Super Cancer Fighters

Proven Natural Remedies That Supplement Mainstream Cancer Treatments

BILL BODRI, M.S.

DISCLAIMER

This book is published under First Amendment rights. Parties involved in providing this book and its contents are not doctors and therefore have no medical background or training. Statements within have not been evaluated by the U.S. Food and Drug Administration or any other medical organization. Before you use anything mentioned in this book, please consult with your physician.

The information in this book is for educational purposes only and designed to provide helpful information on the subjects discussed. This book is not to be considered medical advice in any way, shape or form nor is it a substitute for medical advice. It is not intended as a prescription for treatment nor should it be used to diagnose, treat, cure or prevent any disease. Again, the information contained herein is *not medical advice* and is not intended to replace the care, advice and attention of your personal physician or other health care professionals whom you should always consult for medical treatments. For the diagnosis, treatment or care of any medical condition, consult your own physician.

The author, publisher, editors and others connected with this book do not suggest, endorse, or imply in any way any product/company, treatment, protocol, therapy or cure for any ailment or disease. Nothing within this publication should be considered a "cancer cure." Please consult your health care provider before beginning any new health program, diet, therapy, supplement or health protocol. The reader should regularly consult a physician in matters relating to their health condition and particularly in respect to any symptoms that may require diagnosis or medical attention.

The author, publisher, editors and others connected with this book are not responsible for, nor accept any responsibility over, the content or use of this information. They make no representations concerning the efficacy, appropriateness, or suitability of any of the products, therapies, treatments, protocols or regimens discussed or referenced. The entire risk as to use of this book is assumed by the user. The author, publisher, editors and others connected with this book disclaim responsibility for any adverse effects resulting directly or indirectly from the information contained in this book and are not liable for any damages or negative consequences from any treatment, therapy, protocol, action, application or preparation to any person reading or using the information in this book. In view of the possibility of human error, no party involved in providing this information warrants that the information contained herein is in any respect accurate or complete and they are not responsible nor liable for any errors or omissions that may be found in this book or for the results obtained from the use of such information.

Although many alternative medical treatments have been successfully used for many years, they are often not practiced by conventional medicine and are therefore not "approved" and legal (in some states) for medical professionals to prescribe for their patients, but it is legal for individuals to use them at their own discretion. It therefore becomes necessary to include the following disclaimer: *The offerings made by this publication are to be carefully considered by the user. All responsibility regarding the use of alternative treatments rests with the patient. The author, publisher, editors and others connected with this book do not endorse, recommend or design any specific regimen, therapy or protocol for therapeutic purposes. The decision to use any type of product, protocol or therapy mentioned is entirely your own responsibility. If you have doubts regarding the products and therapies discussed, rely on your doctor's advice. Just because a treatment listed is said to work does not mean it will work for you, and just because it normally produces no side effects does not mean that will be the case for you. Most alternative, complementary, or supplemental cancer therapies/treatments only work on a minority of the people who try them.*

Once again, this book is not to be considered medical advice, which should be sought from a doctor for an accurate medical diagnosis and before the use of any therapy or course of treatment, including the materials discussed. This book merely provides relevant educational information, laid out in front of you so that you can make more informed choices about all your treatment options, the state of your health and well-being. What you do with that information is your choice and your responsibility, and you are always advised to work with your physician.

Top Shape Publishing LLC
1135 Terminal Way Suite 209
Reno, Nevada 89502

ISBN-13: 978-0615880143
ISBN-10: 0615880142

ACKNOWLEDGEMENTS

Part of the reason I wrote this book was because my teacher passed away from cancer. Had I previously known about these various therapies and potential cancer cures, I am positive that the outcome of his condition would have turned out to be entirely different. I am hoping that the benefits of this research, which have been condensed into a highly useable form, can now help others send their cancer into remission. I am fully convinced that in order to beat cancer you should do some additional things on your own other than just the mainstream cancer therapies, and so I've brought that information together to help you (and your physician) tip the odds in your favor.

Tremendous thanks go out to all the people who contributed to the production of this book, which I am truly hoping will help cancer sufferers everywhere.

Mitchell Houston and John Atkinson deserve a thousand kowtows for their painstaking efforts at editing. In particular, John Atkinson made himself into a hero by not only spending a great deal of time trying to make my thoughts conform to the Queen's English, but by also nudging me to include some other pertinent naturopathic details that might help readers who want to seriously pursue various nutritional approaches to cancer.

John Newtson, with his excellent copywriting skills, put on his thinking cap to come up with the book title that he felt would correctly summarize the book's contents. Lastly, I must also thank my graphic artist, Steve Amarillo, for the wonderful job he did on the cover graphics.

CONTENTS

PREFACE

Many newly diagnosed cancer patients think, "I trust my doctor to do everything he needs to do so that I get well." However, they rarely ask, "What else can I be doing on my own, with my own efforts, to get well? What can I do at home that will aid the effectiveness of his therapies?"

There are many additional things you can do, beyond just your doctor's basic treatments, to help beat cancer. Primary of all is to change your diet for the better. You must avoid the foods which feed cancer and interfere with your immune system, and switch to a diet which feeds the healthy normal cells of your body.

Second, you have to understand something extremely important, and then act accordingly. In many U.S. states, your doctor is *not allowed* to recommend or prescribe anything other than surgery, chemotherapy or radiation to help you. That's right! Doctors cannot recommend anything else … nada, zip, nothing. In many states it is a felony to even talk about any other alternative treatments. Therefore they probably won't mention any adjunctive aids you might use to help yourself even though they might help save your life. Their medical license may be on the line or they might face jail time if they do.

It's not their fault that they are wrapped up in a legal straightjacket. If you have time, you can read books like *Alive and Well: One Doctor's Experience with Nutrition in the Treatment of Cancer Patients* (Dr. Philip Binzel) to understand this issue better, such as how government agencies and other legal or medical entities will harass doctors who achieve fantastic cancer cure rates by no longer relying on just traditional mainstream cancer treatments. They certainly exist, but you won't normally hear about them.

With so many threats hanging over a physician's head, don't expect them to mention any other beneficial things you can and should do for your condition even though they may know of them. You will have to discover these things on your own, which you are doing with this book in hand. Importantly, don't be surprised that these supplemental aids are out there, for they definitely are! It's just that these therapies have not come into the mainstream yet. Sometimes your oncologist will even say that they don't even want to know about them even if they see them helping you.

Oncologists know exactly how to play the game of ignorance to preserve their livelihood. You have to understand this. Doctors want to help you and they have devoted many years of their lives with this ideal in mind. They will usually do all that they legally can for you, but there are strict guidelines they must follow on what they can legally say and do, and sometimes ignorance on their part protects both of you. When you think this through, it should become obvious that there are almost certainly very many other beneficial practices that you can use for cancer that they simply cannot suggest, which are the ones you are about to learn.

The best thing you can do, therefore, is to consult an integrative physician, cancer clinic or experienced health coach when you get cancer to obtain additional opinions of any extra help you can give yourself to get well. You should consult someone who is not subject to the legal risks of conventional doctors and who has used many beneficial therapies besides mainstream cancer treatments. Yes, there are such therapies that have been *well proven* through many scientific studies and authoritative clinical experience as you shall soon see.

In fact, many alternative cancer treatments often have a 40% to 50% cure rate for *advanced* cancer patients, which is far beyond that of mainstream therapies. Sometimes cure rates as high as 90% can be attained if patients start using integrative cancer therapies immediately rather than turn to them after their mainstream therapies fail. Therefore when looking for a second or even third medical opinion on your condition, you should certainly consult an integrative physician, especially when you know that many orthodox cancer treatments often have less than a 3% "cure rate."

Now, if you want to stick to just the mainstream cancer therapies offering the highest chances of success for your condition, your best chances of using the right therapy will come from visiting the most renowned cancer treatment centers possible that are the most advanced in terms of staying up-to-date with the most current research. These are usually the only ones that will know which treatments will work best for certain types of cancer, such as which chemotherapy agents typically work best for the particular mutations in your own tumor's genes. They will also often know which orthodox therapies would be of little use for your cancer, so that they wouldn't necessarily recommend chemotherapy if your cancer doesn't normally respond to this treatment. Once again, for the best mainstream treatments you should go to the most up-to-date cancer center possible.

As to integrative physicians, they typically combine a number of different holistic, naturopathic protocols that aim to block cancer's many possible survival routes, whilst simultaneously trying to attack it from multiple angles. They use treatments that also aim to clean up the various problems that might have caused cancer in the first place. They typically try to address your biochemical imbalances and systemic dysfunctions, work to bolster your immune system, try to help repair the DNA replication process, replenish missing nutrients, remove toxicity from your body, attack the cancer directly and so on. Hence they often use entirely different strategies than the mainstream trio of just chemotherapy, surgery and radiation that most doctors must legally adhere to.

Unfortunately, while many of the highly effective therapies used by integrative physicians will increase your chances of beating cancer, reduce the side effects of the mainstream therapies and/or make those same therapies much more effective, you will probably never hear of them from an ordinary oncologist. It is not that these options don't exist or are not available. It is not that they are unproven and don't work. It is just that an ordinary oncologist doesn't know about them or isn't allowed to use them or recommend them, and for various reasons they aren't actively promoted by the FDA, pharmaceutical companies and the media.

If your oncologist is not an integrative physician (a practitioner of alternative, complementary medicine who combines treatments in this fashion), you will be out of luck in having your medical regimen embody this approach unless you research to discover what some of these supplemental therapies are on your own and then use them. Many can certainly be combined with traditional cancer treatments to reduce their side effects and make them more effective. This is what the integrative physicians try to do, and it's best to go to one directly or to a clinic offering such possibilities. But if you cannot, then finding the most powerful supplemental therapies that are easy to use on your own will require some extensive research, just when you might not have much time available to do so. The reason that this book was written was to help you get started immediately on this process of education and action.

The truth is that cancer patients will usually fare much better with integrative therapies, and their conventional treatments will work better if used in conjunction with supplemental naturopathic therapies. This could mean something as simple as drinking green tea, or doing a weekly coffee enema to help detox your body of the dying cells being released into your bloodstream because of cancer treatments. There are many easy, supplemental things you can do at home that will help you fight cancer, support your immune system, improve your quality of life and more.

Unfortunately, most people never bother to get a second opinion about their cancer to discover these things, but upon their diagnosis immediately rush into chemotherapy, surgery or radiation protocols even though these avenues might not be best for them. If you feel you are being rushed into such a decision without being given time to investigate your various alternatives, you should stop and ponder the underlying issues carefully.

In any case, once you find out that you have cancer, shouldn't you then start taking any readily available natural agents that are synergistic with other therapies and which will help produce better treatment outcomes? Even if your doctor doesn't mention them, do you honestly think there are absolutely no supplemental therapies that are perfectly compatible with conventional treatment options? Of course there are! At worst you are just wasting some money if you use some of these inexpensive options. Your life is at stake, so why not? If something doesn't hurt, can possibly help, and only costs money, wouldn't that be something you'd want to know about? That's why this book was born!

If this common sense perspective appeals to you, and many would argue that it should, this book will make your task of discovering some of those supplemental therapies much easier. Several of the most effective, inexpensive and simple alternative therapies covered can be combined with all sorts of conventional therapies to dramatically improve their results, and many have even been used on their own to eliminate cancer. Common sense once again suggests that when your life is at stake, you should be doing everything possible to get well. This means using multiple approaches for cancer that attacks it from different angles because you don't want to stake everything on a single therapy or approach and then later find out that it didn't work, thus losing valuable time in the process.

There is absolutely no animosity to mainstream medicine here, but there is a big emphasis on *personal wisdom and common sense*. You are reminded to become a very informed patient and then, after weighing up all your options, rely on your own decision making process since it is *your life* that is at stake, not theirs. People with cancer should be able to choose the treatments they want. They should be allowed to hedge their bets by using supplemental therapies in addition to mainstream treatments. It makes sense to use proven, extra methods that might help save your life which you can easily combine with orthodox cancer treatments to get better results. It makes sense to help yourself as much as possible since your life is at stake. It makes sense to use supplemental aids that have been known to cure people of cancer on their own.

For instance, if you are going to undergo chemotherapy, why wouldn't you want to do something extra that your doctor hasn't recommended but which will stop it from destroying your immune system and turning you into a walking zombie? There are many supplementary therapies that can complement conventional cancer treatments quite well along these lines, and integrative physicians have been using them for decades because of their excellent results. But do you know about them?

With that objective of education in mind, this book will introduce some of the most important adjunctive therapies possible to help you get started with your healing challenge.

1
INTRODUCTION

One hundred years ago, only one out of every thirty-three individuals got cancer in the United States. Today nearly half of the population will get cancer. In fact, cancer has become the leading cause of death in the United States. However, a cancer diagnosis does not have to be your death sentence. Many people have eliminated cancer and completely gotten well by doing just a little more than what mainstream medicine asks, which means taking some health matters into your own hands.

You maximize your chances for beating cancer by becoming an informed patient who fully evaluates *all* your treatment options, and who therefore looks beyond just the traditional mainstream cancer therapies. One thing that you shouldn't do is to simply put your life entirely in the hands of the mainstream medical establishment without also educating yourself to discover all the various other options available to you. You should always seek a second or third opinion for any health condition and cancer is no exception. You should seek consultations with doctors who use different medical approaches and never just let the health establishment handle all your medical decisions without being an active participant in the process.

Because your life is at stake, you should not unquestioningly do whatever somebody else asks but should apply very careful consideration to *all* of your various cancer treatment options, even those that belong to the field of "alternative," "complementary," "integrative," "naturopathic" or "holistic" medicine. This includes determining whether you want to use any extra therapies at home to help your odds of beating cancer. When you understand what your cancer physician will do and how it is supposed to work, it is important to also ask how you can also help yourself at home.

If you are to succeed at beating cancer, it is first necessary to clearly understand your actual odds of survival when you are going to use any of the therapies that traditional doctors might recommend. Specifically, you need to become an educated patient and know how effective those therapies might be for your type of cancer. You also need to understand the typical side effects of those treatments and how often they occur.

This information will help you decide what to do next because you may discover that the odds are not in your favor if you use certain therapies, or that the side effects can be so horrendously debilitating that other treatment options should also be considered. In the medical field, there is a well-known saying that your treatment may kill you before your cancer does! You will therefore find that many traditional cancer doctors might not choose for themselves the very same treatments they are recommending to patients because of a joint consideration of their side effects and efficacy. Thoughts should start running through your head, "Why should I do something painful and debilitating if, at best, it just adds about two months to my life?"

Fighting cancer takes a great deal of effort and commitment, which can only come when you fully realize the gravity of your situation so as to become fully committed to your various treatment options. For instance, many cancer self-treatments fail because the patient starts using them too late, and then doesn't have the energy, willpower and commitment to continue following a detailed regimen to recover. Also, many won't give up their lifestyle factors which continue to enable the cancer.

Now if you know your odds of survival and the cure rates for the mainstream medical therapies that have been proposed, it will be far easier to decide what to do, such as whether to apply some additional supplemental therapies on your own that your doctors wouldn't normally recommend. To illustrate this, let's examine the topic of chemotherapy. Oncologists typically use chemotherapy as a main treatment of choice even though its efficacy for treating most cancers is minimal. Don't believe this statement? Go to the internet right now and look up "The Contribution of

Cytotoxic Chemotherapy to 5-year Survival in Adult Malignancies," by Graeme Morgan, Robyn Ward and Michael Barton. Clinical Oncology (2004) 16: 549-560.

This study looked at over 150,000 chemotherapy cases from 1990 to 2004 for many different types of cancer, and concluded: "The overall contribution of curative and adjuvant cytotoxic chemotherapy to 5-year survival in adults was estimated to be 2.3% in Australia and 2.1% in the USA." For example, if a total of 72,903 patients received chemotherapy, and after five-years only 1690 of them were still alive, then only 2.3% of them benefitted from chemotherapy. Therefore the "contribution of chemotherapy to five-year survival" is only 2.3%. This five-year survival rate is basically the fraction of people who survived after undergoing chemotherapy, which shows how useful it is.

The authors, two of whom are radiation oncologists and the other a practicing professor of medical oncology, concluded "chemotherapy only makes a minor contribution to cancer survival." In other words, for many types of cancer, *chemotherapy gives very little survival benefit*. It certainly does help in many types of cancer, which is why it is often considered the best course of treatment, but before using it you should get the facts from your doctor to make sure that it helps with *your type of cancer*. You don't want your doctor recommending ineffective and painful chemotherapy treatments just so he can say he "did something."

This study showed that chemotherapy only contributes about 2-3% to cancer cures. Some have argued that this number should be 5-6% or even 8%, but even then *the message is still the same*. In fact, chemotherapy was found to provide few benefits at all to soft tissue sarcomas, skin melanomas and cancers of the uterus, prostate, bladder, kidney, multiple melanoma and pancreas. Thus, make sure the statistics show that it helps with your type of cancer before you use it because it is commonly given to most cancer patients even though it only helps a limited minority. Not much has changed for most cancers since 1985 when John Cairns, professor of microbiology at Harvard University, stated in *Scientific American*: "Aside from certain rare cancers, it is not possible to detect any sudden changes in death rates for any of the major cancers that could be credited for chemotherapy. Whether any of the common cancers can be cured by chemotherapy has yet to be established."

Unless you have one of the types of cancer that responds to chemotherapy in a highly beneficial way (such as Hodgkin's disease, testicular cancer, etc.), or the medical community starts using chemotherapy in a more targeted manner (such as with IPT Insulin Potentiation Therapy, where tumors are also sensitivity tested to determine which chemotoxic agent would be most effective), the actual numbers show that it usually won't help much at all. However, it will definitely poison your body and depress your immune system at the very time when you want the exact opposite to be happening. It is so toxic that it can actually shorten your life, and sometimes people die from the chemotherapy rather than the cancer.

ASK YOUR DOCTOR

This is why when any cancer therapy is proposed to you, you must ask your doctor the following questions:

- Since cancer "response rates" (which only refer to short term tumor shrinkage) are not the same as "recovery rates" (where the individual becomes cancer-free), what are the chances that this therapy will help me become cancer free and live longer than five years?
- Since some cancer treatments can cause potentially fatal complications, what is the estimated fatality rate for the treatments you are recommending?
- Is this a treatment meant to *cure me*, or is it just a treatment being administered in hopes of prolonging life? If it is just to help prolong my life, how much does it usually extend the lifespan?
- What are *all* the side effects of this treatment, and what will this treatment do to my quality of life? What percentage of patients experience each side effect (since side effects are known, the percentages will be definitely known)? What medications are prescribed for those side effects, and what are the side effects of those medications?
- What are the chances that cancer will come back if these treatments are a success?

- Even if you help cure me with your therapy, what else will you do to address my *systemic condition,* which is the root cause of the disease, so that the cancer doesn't come back?

Your quality of life, life expectancy and whether you are addressing the causes of your cancer are all important issues you need to consider when evaluating various treatment options. We should all beware of medical treatments that create a great deal of suffering (or cost a lot of money, thus draining your bank account) but which do not address the roots of the problem or prolong life in any significant way.

For instance, very often you will find cancer patients who immediately underwent surgery to "cut out" their tumor, or who underwent painful chemotherapy or radiation, only to find that it "came back" months later since this approach never addressed the root causes of their cancer. You cannot just cut out someone's tumor and say, "you are cured." Think about it: will removing tumors in itself prevent your body from growing more tumors? If your underlying systemic condition is not treated as well, shouldn't you expect tumors to form again? You cannot simply "cut cancer out" and expect it to be gone if all the factors that allowed it to develop still remain in your body afterwards. You should not assume you have removed its causes unless you change your diet, lifestyle and everything that might have previously contributed to its growth and development.

The tumor is only the outward sign of an underlying systemic problem that must be corrected, and how long you go without more tumors developing again will have everything to do with whether you make positive changes in your life that will transform your internal biochemistry for the better. What will your doctor do to help you transform your inner terrain? Since he won't do anything at all, that's why you should look into many of these supplemental therapies. They will help along these and many other lines.

People rarely bother to ask common sense questions such as, "How will cutting out the tumor fix my immune system?" or "What else must I do to rid my body of cancer and get well?" You must certainly address the underlying factors that led to cancer in the first place to truly get well and stay well, which is why I suggest you always ask for a "second opinion" from a holistic, complementary, naturopathic or integrative physician. Call him or her what you will, but you should seek a medical opinion from another perspective that will address the underlying causes of your cancer's development and progression.

If you want to know the typical survival rates after diagnosis for various types of cancer, you can find them in John Boik's book, *Cancer and Natural Medicine*. Dr. Lorraine Day (DrDay.com) has a DVD called "Cancer Doesn't Scare Me Anymore," which also reveals the side effects and real cure rates of most cancer treatments. Sometimes you can also find these statistics on the web, but it usually requires much digging. It doesn't matter where they are; you must find them for your condition.

Cancer researcher Ralph Moss has also revealed much of this information in his various books, such as *Questioning Chemotherapy*. These numbers, which doctors won't always tell you, will help you determine just how aggressive you must be in pursuing alternative therapies *other* than just those proposed by the traditional medical establishment. You may find that the odds of success for the mainstream therapies proposed for your condition are so poor that logic *screams* that extra supplemental effort is required or an entirely different course of medical treatment is needed than what is suggested.

Make no mistake about it: many mainstream therapies are excellent for cancer and sometimes surgery, chemotherapy and radiation are exactly the treatments a cancer patient needs and should use. You certainly don't want to be entirely antagonistic toward these options. However, sometimes various integrative therapies will offer much better hope, and it is your job to find this out *sooner rather than later* before all your money is used up and your body has become so damaged by mainstream treatments that even integrative therapies will have a hard time helping you to heal. Since a traditional oncologist doesn't usually know anything about integrative therapies, you should always try to go to a cancer clinic or integrative oncologist for this valuable second opinion.

It would be better for cancer patients to get the right treatments at the start rather than have to use supplemental therapies at home to protect themselves or supercharge their traditional therapies so that they are much more effective. However, because doctors are not using all the cutting edge testing that is available, they are simply not selecting treatments on the basis of their effectiveness and thus this extra help is required. Without extra help, the odds of survival for most traditional cancer treatments are usually very poor.

Once again, if the odds of survival for your type of cancer aren't good, it certainly makes a great deal of sense to get extra supplemental help outside of the traditional medical treatment path. *Furthermore, you should get started at those things as early as possible once you have been diagnosed*, before any mainstream therapies have a chance to destroy your immune system completely and weaken your body to the verge of collapse, at which point even integrative therapies might not be able to help.

It would be *unwise to wait* until after mainstream therapies fail before you start using safe supplemental therapies since orthodox cancer treatments often allow cancer to spread while severely damaging your body in the process. In dealing with cancer, you want all the help you can get from the start and sometimes it is the extra things you do that will help you put your cancer into remission. You want to start on those things *earlier rather than later*, especially while your body is still strong and your immune system is still functioning.

There are countless non-mainstream therapies that certainly won't hurt you, and which many integrative physicians have successfully used to produce hundreds of thousands of cancer cures, even though the traditional medical establishment won't even look at them or recommend them. Change happens slowly in the medical community, *especially when great sums of money are at risk of being lost when things change*, so it is up to you to go outside the box to find these other things that can help you and possibly save your life. Only after many years will you ever see these therapies adopted by the mainstream institutions. It will eventually happen, but you cannot wait for the slow process of adoption because you are sick *now*.

With your life at stake, you shouldn't be afraid to try some safe supplemental therapies or avoid them because you want to please your doctors. Since an alternative physician may very well fully embrace those same therapies, you should make your decision on whether to use extra therapies after personal research and consideration. Furthermore, which is extremely important, *you should make any decisions on which therapies to use at home* rather than in a hospital setting or in any doctor's office when you are feeling all sorts of pressure.

It is certainly smart thinking to add supplemental, adjunctive therapies to your life, which won't hurt you and may actually even cure you, especially when they are known to have helped hundreds of thousands of people despite the lack of a "blessing" from the mainstream establishment. What is the harm in using these optional aids, especially when they are fully employed in many other locations by skilled physicians, too? The only potential loss is the fact that you might be spending your own money on something that naysayers claim is a useless placebo. If that's so, why not since it won't hurt? With so much at stake, you should not feel held back from using helpful supplemental remedies or alternative therapies simply because they have not yet been incorporated into mainstream medicine.

If you think I haven't made my case because of a lack of evidence, let me show you, with three simple examples, how slow the mainstream cancer medical community can be in adopting methods that might save your life.

First of all, there are now modern chemo-sensitivity tests for tumors that can tell you which chemotherapy agent has the highest likelihood of success in eliminating your cancer, but most oncologists don't know about them or will not use them. These testing possibilities include the:

- BioFocus test available in Germany (Biofocus.de)
- Research Genetic Cancer Center (RGCC) test available in Greece (Rgcc-genlab.com)
- Rational Therapeutics (Rational-t.com) Ex Vivo Apoptotic Assay developed by Dr. Robert Nagoumey
- Weisenthal Cancer Group testing (Weisenthalcancer.com)

Now that you know that these tests are available, it would almost be a crime to undergo chemotherapy treatments without insisting that your tumor was first tested to see which chemotherapy agents would be the most effective for your cancer! There is an extremely high probability that the chemotoxic agent the doctor selects may not work at all for your diagnosis, and yet oncologists will rarely use any tests to determine which agents have the highest chances of actually working. What's wrong with this picture?

Since chemotherapy drugs are *only effective 30% of the time when they are selected based on clinical trials,* you should insist that the chemicals your doctor uses are selected with as much certainty as possible for your condition. Without testing, the odds are against you that your doctors will use the most effective agents possible. You should want your oncologist to avoid using ineffective therapies and develop the best treatment plan from the start, so why don't mainstream physicians use these tests?

Furthermore, often your body will develop Multiple Drug Resistant (MDR) cells that chemotherapy cannot kill, whereas some alternative therapies can. A biopsy that is tested for MDR cells will tell you the percentage of the tumor upon which chemotherapy will have no effect. Why doesn't your doctor test for this?

Secondly, there is also a cancer treatment option called "IPT insulin potentiation therapy" (see *Treating Cancer with Insulin Potentiation Therapy* by Dr. Ross Hauser), which allows chemotherapy doses to be reduced to 1/10 of normal. This allows chemotherapy to more accurately target cancer cells without a patient suffering the major debilitating side effects for which chemotherapy is known. It is rapidly growing in popularity, yet most doctors don't use it either. Why wouldn't you want your tumor to be first genetically tested to see which chemotherapy agent would be the most effective against it, and then use *that* chemical in greatly reduced dosages that have the same efficacy, or better, while reducing the known harmful side effects of the treatments?

Third, it is strange that many oncologists will never even warn you against eating sugar, which actually *feeds cancer to make it stronger*. Paradoxically, they will often dissuade you from using a few supplements or dietary changes that will supercharge their therapies rather than interfere with them. They may warn you away from the very things that have countless scientific studies proving their effectiveness for beating cancer and which have frequently produced "spontaneous cancer remissions" just by themselves. You'll have to figure out the reasons for all these oversights on your own. All I can say is that you should always seek a second and third doctor's opinion for your treatments to make sure mistakes and oversights don't happen.

Once again, when a smart cancer patient looks at all the survival statistics, they will quickly realize that the wrong approach to getting well is to blindly say, "Radiate me, cut me open, give me chemo. I'm not going to challenge you by asking any questions. I'm not going to participate in any decision-making that involves my life. I'm not going to educate myself about my entire set of treatment options. I trust you completely to use the most effective therapies for my cancer. Just do anything you want."

This is often a recipe for death. Common sense dictates that you need to do more for yourself and your family. People are depending on you and so by using some wisdom you can become extremely proactive against cancer to help beat it. If you do nothing then already you know what your future will be with 100% certainty. Only if you do something will you have a chance to change that future.

If you want to beat cancer, you absolutely must become more informed. You must decide to take some personal responsibility for your cure, rather than surrender all that responsibility to others. You should start doing some supplemental, additional things at home right *now* before it becomes even more difficult to reverse your condition because you may have become too weakened by your cancer or orthodox treatment prescriptions.

You certainly should do some things on your own to maximize your chances of getting well, but traveling this road means that you must first do some investigation to see what additional non-mainstream approaches can help you to get well. There are many simple, easy self-help therapies used by advanced cancer clinics all over the world that are well proven, but which the mainstream medical establishment has not adopted yet.

Some supplemental therapies can attack cancer cells directly and kill them. Some supplemental protocols can help to revert cancer cells back into normal cells. Some have the potential to shrink tumors extremely quickly. Some aids will prevent cachexia, give you energy or make your body stronger. This will "buy you time" for other therapies (whether mainstream or not) to work at beating the cancer. Some supplemental aids will strengthen your body's detoxification system so that it can deal with all the toxins and cellular debris being generated by your other therapies. All sorts of helpful supplemental aids are available that work through different mechanisms.

Since you often don't have a lot of time to get going, you don't need a book thick with lots of useless information that doesn't get you to the point of actually doing anything that will help you. Many cancer books are filled with all sorts of interesting facts that produce an overload of extraneous information that can paralyze you from taking any concrete positive steps that will move you to getting well. This book is not like that.

Other books might be interesting, informative and even entertaining, but you need to get on with doing something other than just more reading. You should not be focused on collecting knowledge over taking action. You need to be taking positive action now. You should be immediately focused on taking helpful steps to get well. After learning something, you should focus on immediately *implementing what you learn*. Specifically, you should focus on constructing a logical, clear plan to get well and then immediately and consistently start *working that plan to beat cancer*.

We will therefore focus on some of the simplest extra things you can do at home that will have the most impact by either directly eliminating cancer, by helping your other therapies to work many times better, or by helping you to feel better and buying you extra time. Several hundred therapies have been considered and this book focuses on just a small subset of the most effective ones that can usually stand on their own. They are self-help therapies that you can do at home which usually don't interfere with mainstream cancer regimens, but which commonly supercharge their effectiveness.

Many of these supplemental aids will give you more energy, help eliminate pain, make you stronger or help you feel better. Many of these helpmates have even cured people of cancer just by themselves, but you should not think of them as "cancer cures." They are to be considered "adjunctive," "supplemental," "additional," "extra," "optional" aids to any other cancer treatment regimens, especially the mainstream cancer therapies that often put a strain on your body. Most are not contraindicated by mainstream orthodox treatments but they can very often help to dramatically improve your traditional therapy results dramatically.

Basically, whether you want to remain wholly dependent on traditional conventional cancer therapies or not, many of these adjunctive aids will assist your health in various ways and can very often buy you more time so that your other cancer treatments can work. This is especially important when you are in stage IV or when you have an aggressive cancer condition. However, one shouldn't make the mistake of waiting until their cancer is late stage and only then start using helpful supplemental therapies. Once you've been diagnosed with cancer, since you know the final outcome you want to attack it from different angles with everything you've got, while still relatively healthy, so it doesn't have time to adapt and grow stronger.

A major principle of complementary medicine is that you must protect and strengthen your healthy cells during this time because they are the ones that will keep you alive. Their condition determines how long you will have to treat your cancer. You can certainly support your healthy non-cancerous cells through a better diet and with special supplements, but a typical oncologist usually doesn't know how to advise you along these lines or will often tell you to avoid supplements altogether during chemotherapy.

Even so, your first priority at home is to nourish the normal cells of your body that will keep you alive and help reduce the toxicity caused by cancer treatments and/or the lysing of cancer cells flooding your system. Since mainstream therapies will not do this, you can use some supplemental helpmates on your own that will nourish your body's healthy cells and help keep all of your body's functional systems in tiptop shape. This is very important because of the damage that orthodox treatments can inflict on your body. Think about this for a moment and logic should tell you that this makes perfect sense.

These are just a few reasons why these supplemental therapies are so important. To help yourself heal, you should get started on some of them right away. Even for those of you who are reading this book and who don't have any cancer, the dietary advice in particular will not only help prevent cancer in the first place but will improve your health and make you stronger. Furthermore, by learning about these therapies and dietary choices now, you will have a bigger arsenal of weapons against all sorts of health disorders, even though we are obviously concentrating on just cancer.

As stated, most of these approaches do not interfere with traditional therapies, which is why they are called supplemental or "adjunctive," meaning that you can do them alongside of traditional therapies. "Adjunctive" means an additional substance, therapy, treatment, protocol or procedure that increases the efficacy or safety of a primary medical procedure. This is exactly what many of these protocols do.

You should know that there are plenty of integrative physicians who make these proven therapies the *core part* of their treatment protocols for healing patients of cancer. The most effective integrative oncologists will combine several different therapies together, for their synergistic benefits, to maximize your chances of recovery. Their overall protocol will very often include some of the very therapies that we are about to discuss.

If you want to pursue the most effective complementary anti-cancer protocols, you should definitely turn to expert integrative doctors and health practitioners. They will typically combine a variety of diverse approaches to your condition because this is what normally produces the best success rates. Most alternative cancer therapies are not strong enough by themselves and often don't work fast enough in cases of advanced cancer, so the best strategy for healing is to combine several different therapeutic approaches together. This book will thus help you to answer the burning question, "What more can I do on my own along these lines that will help my situation for the better?"

Now because complicated protocols require the help and guidance of cancer experts, we are only going to concentrate on *the simplest adjunctive cancer therapies* because we want to focus on what you can immediately do in terms of self-help. This book does not include protocols that must be performed by a physician, such as intravenous injections, hypothermia and bio-oxidative therapies. It excludes powerful electro-medicine protocols that involve expensive equipment which most people cannot afford. Even though you don't need a physician's help for the supplemental aids covered, which can be as simple as drinking a cup of green tea, you are strongly advised to run these various therapies by your doctors or other health experts in order to gain from their judicious opinions and helpful guidance.

Work with them. Many will respect you for doing your research, adopting a fighting spirit and being proactive in trying to beat cancer. Many health professionals are fully aware of the benefits of such adjunctive measures and want to learn more such as how to best implement them, even though they cannot say so or cannot use them. By working with your health expert and making it clear that you are determined to do your bit, you may even end up helping the medical establishment to incorporate these therapies, even though it is slow to change its standard range of procedures. Your attitude and behavior may even help pave the way for others in the future.

Physicians usually have some of the best ethics of all professions. In the United States, 98% of medical students swear some kind of vow based on the Hippocratic oath, which incorporates the ideals of honesty and justice in their practice. Even though their hands may be tied towards using some complementary therapies, they may well tacitly approve of them. Physicians want you to get well. All their years of study have this admirable purpose in mind. If you somehow feel that your doctor doesn't care or doesn't want you to get well but just sees you as a source of income, then that is another issue entirely and a reason to look for an alternative doctor. These types of people are extremely rare, however, and the medical establishment has its own mechanisms for preventing and dealing with this behavior.

The short of it is this: when you are diagnosed with cancer, often you won't have much time to investigate many different therapies that might be beneficial. However, because the clock is ticking you should immediately get started at various highly helpful adjunctive therapies right away, and you need to know what these high priority options are. You should be seeking therapies that you can immediately do at home, which will help to eliminate cancer all on their own and/or "supercharge" the results of your other treatments. That cuts down on all the options you need consider.

If that is your line of thinking then this book is perfect for you. It is for people who want to do more than just hope, wait and see. It is for people who are doing nothing at all and want to do something. It's for people who are already doing chemo, radiation or surgery and who want to do more. It's for people who are doing integrative treatments and want to do more. It's also for people who may have been abandoned by the medical establishment, such as those given a very poor prognosis and sent home to die in a more comfortable environment, but who don't want to give up hope. These individuals especially need to know that various adjunctive therapies can often extend your life and just might save you. It's for people in remission who want to prevent a cancer recurrence. It's also for people who never had cancer, but who want to prevent it from ever happening.

With precious time at stake, often your head will be spinning after hearing the cancer diagnosis and you won't have the time to evaluate the hundreds of nutraceutical supplements, cancer diet options, and other supplemental regimens available. Nevertheless, you still need to get started at doing something highly impactful that will probably help but won't hurt. This book is for you. It is designed to immediately get you doing something beneficial for your healing.

Mainstream medical professionals may tell you that these adjunctive cancer therapies are unproven or that they don't work, but that just isn't true. Research them on the internet and you'll find thousands of successful case studies, testimonials, research reports, clinical trials and so on. In becoming a health detective, you will often find a clear history that this positive information has been suppressed because the approach threatens the financial interests of the medical industry and its vested interests.

The truth is that the supplemental therapies you are about to learn have been used by countless physicians and cancer survivors. Often they have produced complete cures on their own even though they are just supplemental aids. You should not count on any single approach "curing" anyone, however, but you should also weigh the common sense consideration in your mind that runs, "It might help. If it makes sense and doesn't hurt but can help, then why not? It's only my money. What is that compared to my life?"

For your best chances of reversing cancer to get well, you certainly should take some healing matters into your own hands, such as your diet and supportive nutrition or supplements. You must transform your inner terrain to improve its current condition. An ordinary oncologist is in all likelihood not trained to give you any helpful advice along these lines, especially when it comes to beneficial diets, nutrition and supplements. Nonetheless, you must consider that the stronger you get from this additional help, the more likely it is that you will then do better with traditional therapies if that is the road you choose to take. With the outcome of cancer treatments so poor and uncertain, why shouldn't everyone be given the freedom of choice to supplement their main treatment regimen with helpful aids like these? Just make sure you clear their usage with a health professional.

I bear zero ill will against traditional orthodox cancer therapies and the mainstream medical establishment. However, I hope everything you choose to do to be as effective as possible, including mainstream treatments. These complementary aids you are about to learn have certainly helped people improve their clinical results tremendously, which is why they are being cited. Just search the internet for more research and you will certainly find individuals who can attest to their effectiveness. They are easy to implement, extremely powerful in many beneficial ways and are inexpensive in most cases. They are the primers of a self-help approach to beating cancer and getting well.

Let's talk about undergoing chemotherapy once again to illustrate some of the points we have been making. The fact is this: studies clearly show that better nutrition improves the results of chemotherapy. Another widely known fact is that chemotherapy hurts your body and destroys your immune system, and many people become sick from its toxicity. Since certain supplements or additional helpmate therapies can protect your body and detoxify your bloodstream of cancer debris while improving the effectiveness of chemotherapy, why wouldn't you want to use them? Certain supplemental therapies can definitely lessen both the dangers and toxicity of chemotherapy and radiation. In some cases, nutritional protocols that involve particular supplements even do a better job at defeating cancer than traditional therapies for certain conditions.

Nevertheless, in spite of the overwhelming evidence supporting special types of beneficial nutrition or the beneficial use of nutritional supplements taken during many forms of cancer treatment, some oncologists will incorrectly say that nutritional supplements are worthless on their own or are contraindicated during chemo and/or radiation therapy. There are hundreds of published medical studies *proving the exact opposite*, and when I was getting my graduate degree in clinical nutrition one of my professors was livid that the medical establishment kept ignoring these facts. If a doctor feeds you this line, ask them to show you the research proving that certain supplements make chemotherapy less effective. You will find they almost certainly cannot show you any, or can show you perhaps one (possibly faulty) study against a hundred that say it helps.

When it comes to cancer, some mainstream oncologists will even go so far as to say that your diet and healthier nutrition is of little importance, too. They may not even tell you that all cancer patients should avoid sugar, which is the main dietary rule that every cancer patient should know.

Doctors usually lack this knowledge because they are not normally trained in curative or supportive nutrition, but you must understand that *your diet is one of the primary factors in being able to survive cancer.* If you continue eating a poor diet, it will undermine both orthodox mainstream cancer therapies and any alternative therapies, too! Poor nutrition, which is entirely your own responsibility, will make healing that much harder.

There are various economic, educational, political, and group-think reasons behind all this ignorance (see Ralph Moss' *The Cancer Industry* for some relevant explanations), but the plain fact is that wrong beliefs together with prejudice will prevent you from receiving some of the most worthwhile information that might save your life unless you research matters for yourself. Ignorance on your part, or possibly even on your doctor's part, may therefore threaten your life.

Don't put yourself in that situation. Become informed because your life is at stake. Go ahead and research any of these supplemental cancer therapies on your own. With just a few keystrokes on Google, you will be able to trace down all sorts of other information about these therapies that the mainstream medical establishment has not yet digested and adopted, but which in time it may well acknowledge. Can you afford to wait until it does so? No. You must get started on extra efforts at healing right away. After all, your life is on the line.

It is another fact that some cancer centers and oncologists are less up-to-date in applying the latest research findings in the field than others. Regardless of the reasons why, therefore once again it is your job to quickly educate yourself on all sorts of alternative integrative and supplementary therapies that might help you beat your cancer, because of the possibility of ignorance within the medical profession, and then apply them. Remember the 80/20 rule: emphasize whatever has the greatest potential impact for your health rather than concentrate on superficial things that promise very little benefit.

You must remember this prioritizing rule because you cannot possibly do everything that is helpful, nor do you want to waste your money, time and efforts by concentrating on minor things that don't produce a great impact. You want to do whatever gives you the biggest bang for your limited resources of effort, time and money. The therapies within this book were chosen precisely because they are high impact aids, so these are the first things to consider.

You would be surprised how many people, after reading a book on alternative cancer therapies, will foolishly ignore this principle and concentrate on something minor (like buying a water purifier) while ignoring everything else, and then think that having done this one tiny thing is going to help them defeat cancer in a big way. This sort of misplaced emphasis is common, and you must simply avoid it.

On the other hand, many at home adjunctive cancer therapies do involve very small things that can definitely have a big impact on your health, including such small changes as drinking fresh vegetable juices rather than milk or sodas. However, as stated, you cannot do all the possibly helpful things in existence. Fighting cancer can be tiring and you probably won't have enough time or energy to do many extra things at all. Nevertheless, you need to know how to get started with a small but extremely smart subset of extra optional things that often help GREATLY.

When others try to dissuade you from such adjunctive therapies, claiming they are useless or ineffective, you have to ask how this can be so if so many others have used them successfully. Whenever you also hear that any of these therapies are dangerous, you should also ask in return, "Oh really? Dangerous compared to what? Chemotherapy?"

As health activist and researcher Gary Null once said after studying the track records of many integrative physicians treating cancer, the best ones used a *combination of all sorts of various alternative therapies*, so many things should be considered. You should search for a doctor who will put together a complete set of supplemental therapies for your mainstream cancer protocols, otherwise you will have to do this on your own. Now is the time to find out which ones can work, which doctors might use them, and then pursue them if the experts you consult think they will benefit you.

To kick cancer into remission, you should immediately start using a combination of the most powerful supplemental aids available, many of which have cured patients even though they are just helpmates. You should immediately start doing extra beneficial protocols before cancer has a chance to spread and before chemo or other mainstream therapies weaken your body so much that your immune system is largely destroyed and unable to recover. Using a combination of several effective therapies that attack cancer from different perspectives, and relying on the principle of multiple redundancy rather than depending on just one approach alone, is the reason why integrative physicians commonly achieve cancer cure rates beating those of the best hospitals and orthodox physicians hands down. Again that's why I strongly urge you to consider some of these approaches.

Before you go in for surgery, chemo or radiation, you should therefore look around and investigate various integrative cancer clinics and physicians and ask for their opinions. You can call some of the health coaches listed in this book or pick up books like *Knockout* (Somers), *Defeat Cancer* (Rowen) or *An Alternative Medicine Definitive Guide to Cancer* (Goldberg) to find the names of integrative clinics and physicians who might help you.

You will find many integrative cancer physicians and clinics that have great success rates because they use a variety of effective approaches to treat cancer that cause far less damage to your body than the typical mainstream protocols. If you have already taken that route, you should certainly discuss some of these supplemental strategies with them, because many have the potential of making your survival odds even better.

The point is that if you actually go and talk to an integrative physician or their patients, you will find that many non-traditional cancer therapies may yield far better results than popular mainstream treatments. Most people don't know this because that information isn't widely publicized, and many doctors don't recognize this either (or they do but are afraid to use these therapies for fear of losing their license). You can definitely find case study after case study of individuals who attribute their survival to alternative therapies that don't follow the normal standards of chemotherapy, radiation and surgery. You just have to do a little research to find this information, so the point is that you cannot immediately dismiss these supplemental approaches as nonsense, as some doctors are wont to do.

Many supplemental aids have definitely produced cancer cures on their own. It only makes sense that if the body can create cancer, it also has the capability of controlling or reversing it given the right kind of support, which is what many of these various complementary, integrative therapies are designed to do with little to no side effects at all.

The gist of it is this: as part of your road back to perfect health again, you should definitely consider using integrative therapies in some form or another. You might also want to use these types of therapies on a maintenance basis to help prevent cancer or its recurrence. There is a clear bias against such therapies in the greater medical community but the plain fact is that they have helped thousands of people in various ways, including by curing cancer. They have *slowly* been creeping into the mainstream tradition and will continue doing so into the future.

Another issue is that these therapies cost very little compared to many mainstream alternatives, which puts the cancer industry at risk of losing tremendous income if they ever became popular. This is just one of the many reasons that the cancer industry tries to suppress them and, having lost sight of its higher calling, sadly often persecutes those who might practice them.

Even so, this does not change the fact that as a cancer patient you must make extra efforts to strengthen, cleanse and heal your body during any type of treatments you undergo, and especially during mainstream procedures that may also attack healthy cells in your body and weaken it. It is strange that patients are sometimes discouraged from using any adjunctive protocols that might help their body, while the mainstream procedures recommended often devastate the body and its immune system.

With cancer you are fighting for your life, so this is a time when you should do some serious thinking. Rely on logic and common sense. Should you not get yourself into tiptop shape to fight cancer? Should you not do everything possible to assist your therapy and increase its effectiveness?

Cancer should be looked at as a disease of the whole body and tumors are just a symptom of this larger disease, so it is up to you to work on fixing the rest of your body since your doctor usually won't address this issue. *This is where a real "cancer cure" comes from.* Cancer is an indicator that your body is systemically toxic and your immune system damaged, and tells you that it needs some dramatic changes to get well. Surgery or radiation, by themselves, will not do that and neither will chemotherapy. What does that leave you?

I want you to think deeply about these things. Consider this, also: if your oncologist has just given you several months to live, don't you think you need every bit of nutritional ammunition possible to help you extend that time so you have a chance to get well? Isn't it logical that the stronger you get, the more likely you will do better with traditional mainstream or any other cancer therapies? Don't you think you owe it to yourself to take advantage of any products that might make conventional treatments safer and more effective, and which reduce the toxic effects of these therapies as they are being administered? Shouldn't you be boosting your own self-healing capabilities?

I would be asking myself, "Shouldn't I be treating my whole body and focusing on rejuvenating my whole person rather than just attacking the cancer or its symptoms? In order to reverse cancer, doesn't it make sense to detoxify my body of contributing poisons and try to correct all the affronts to my immune system? Shouldn't I stop focusing on just the tumor but instead concentrate on the multiple causes that have produced this systemic condition? If I cannot eliminate the cancer, is there some way it can be made into a manageable condition so that I can still go on living?"

If you think along these lines, you would come to the conclusion that it is common sense to augment conventional cancer treatments with adjunctive therapies especially since your doctor is not addressing these issues. It makes perfect sense to start using various nutritional substances and approaches that are known to help cancer patients in many ways and which have been known at times to even lead to cures on their own. If you could take them previously, why can't you take them now since they work to correct the very conditions that cause cancer?

People commonly undergo all sorts of toxic mainstream procedures designed to "produce a response" and "shrink tumors" rather than actually address the underlying causes of that cancer. Don't you think you should do something extra to address the underlying systemic damage, even if your doctor doesn't say anything about this or even if your doctor actually discourages any extra adjunctive help along these lines?

Smart cancer survivors are not the ones who take a "wait and see" attitude before deciding what to do along the route of supplemental aid. They get started at the optional extra additional things, which sometimes produce cures on their own, *immediately*. That means *right now*. They don't waste precious time arguing as their immune system continues to get damaged, but immediately start doing whatever will maximize their chances of turning around their condition, even if it goes beyond the typical advice of the medical establishment.

Throughout history it has usually been the case that those who developed the fighting spirit and helped themselves were the ones who survived and thrived, while those who passively relied on others out of blind faith were often the most disappointed. In which group do you want to be?

If you just surrender yourself to the medical establishment without taking some critical health matters into your own hands, it is very likely – in fact assured – that you will miss many beneficial therapies that have been known to produce cancer cures or a much better quality of life and increased longevity. You may be lowering your chances of survival.

Winners at life typically adopt an attitude similar to the following, "I am not going to let myself die. I am going to look at all these treatment options offered, their known chances of success and consequences. I am not going to let anyone immediately push me into chemotherapy, radiation, surgery or anything else. I'm not going to let anyone bully me into a therapy until I'm fully informed. After I'm fully informed, only then am I going to personally select the treatments which I understand are best for me. And regardless of whatever therapy road I choose, I am going to do everything possible on my own in addition to the help of other health professionals to assist in the healing process through supplemental means."

As stated, once you receive a cancer diagnosis, you should know that your life is at stake and that time is on fire. You cannot afford to be passive. You cannot be complacent. You must immediately start working on changing your internal terrain to reverse your condition. To save your life, you should consider doing *extra things* that are not going to hurt you, which have helped many thousands beat cancer, but which, for various reasons are not currently sanctioned by the medical establishment. So what should you do?

START READING

If you have just been diagnosed with cancer and my words do not convince you of the potential value of non-mainstream therapies, you should immediately get a copy of Suzanne Somers' *Knockout: Interviews With Doctors Who Are Curing Cancer*. These interviews will show you that many effective integrative therapy alternatives are available so that you need not rely on just the traditional mainstream therapies alone. In reading it you will clearly see that many successful therapy alternatives exist and that surgery, chemo and radiation are not all that are available to help you get well.

There are also books like *Outsmart Your Cancer* (Tanya Harter Pearce) and *Defeat Cancer: 15 Doctors of Integrative & Naturopathic Medicine Tell You How* (Connie Strasheim) that I also highly recommend. These books give you the names of integrative doctors and clinics, and various integrative therapies that you might also consider using.

All these books inform you about complementary, integrative treatments that work, and tell you about clinics where you can find them. This book can immediately get you started on several safe, proven, supplemental anti-cancer aids you can use at home while you do any of this other research. Don't ever make the mistake of thinking that these therapies are enough on their own, even though for some people that has indeed been the case. To beat cancer you usually need a doctor's assistance.

Cancer-Free: Your Guide to Gentle, Non-toxic Healing (Bill Henderson) and *Cancer: Step Outside the Box* (Ty Bollinger) also contain extremely valuable information on how to beat cancer and get well. These books give full naturopathic protocols you can use, telling you how to maximize your chances of beating cancer and living a full and healthy life.

Helpful internet websites can also introduce a variety of alternative cancer therapies and explain how they work. NaturalCancerTreatments.com and CancerTutor.com are two such examples. However, the best approach to beating cancer is not to go DIY but to find a cancer physician or other expert whom you can work with, who will design an individualized program for you. You might want to consult with an experienced cancer coach, who has dealt with thousands of patients, to help find such a physician.

When you ponder the many alternative cancer therapies listed in these various books and on websites and start to understand how and why they work, you will definitely find yourself inundated with options. How do you organize it all? There are so many options available that most people initially become paralyzed whilst trying to prioritize what to do first or next. As stated, with so very many available options, the risk is that you end up doing little to nothing or just focus on the least impactful supplemental strategies. The brevity of this book is designed to prevent that common mistake.

This book concentrates only on the most powerful adjunctive therapies that you can use for cancer without much supervision and which you can get started at right away. It is a *short list* of the best do-it-yourself supplemental, adjunctive therapies, all of which can normally be used alongside typical cancer treatments. These supplemental measures will not necessarily cure you, but they will usually help in many ways without interfering with or hurting other treatments.

These protocols can make traditional therapies safer, more powerful and more effective, which is why people commonly use them. At worst you and your doctors should consider them just a waste of some of your money, whereas in truth they usually help tremendously, especially since they attack the problem of cancer from angles *usually not addressed by mainstream medicine.* Their usage is entirely up to you, and once again I recommend that you clear their usage with your health practitioner.

A main principle of this book is that you must take personal responsibility for your health to help your body heal using such extra efforts. All things considered, everyone should probably be using some form of supplemental therapies when they have cancer rather than just solely depend on the limited set of mainstream therapies. This could be something as simple as changing your diet to reduce your sugar intake or eat certain foods. The point is that you probably have to go past the minimal advice that mainstream medicine normally tells you.

If you check around you will even find many people who have beaten cancer, who will also tell you that they did so *in spite of the efforts of the medical establishment.* Confirming what I have said, these people developed a fighting spirit, took matters into their own hands and worked to maximize the chances of a cure by doing all sorts of extra things that the medical establishment did not ask of them and in fact sometimes frowned upon. Sometimes this meant turning their back on the mainstream establishment entirely because it had sent them down a road that led to deepening problems rather than healing, and sometimes it meant working alongside the medical establishment by using supplemental therapies as part of a larger set of integrative health protocols.

Your best chances of beating cancer will come from radically changing the way you have been living, detoxifying your body, boosting your immune system and especially by cleaning up your diet. To get well, you must eliminate the causes of biochemical imbalance that caused cancer in the first place and this starts with your diet. You should take the cancer diagnosis as a wake-up call for the need to dramatically change your life, including how you eat and the way you live.

If your oncologist has just given you several months to live, understand that you need every bit of nutritional ammunition you can get to help put cancer at bay while you fight it. Thus we are talking about switching to clean, nutrient-dense, wholesome nutrition. You also owe it to yourself during this time to take advantage of any beneficial nutraceutical supplements that might help your body to heal and extend your life.

Unfortunately, one of the roadblocks to self-help is the fact that most people will not apply what they are taught to do what will help them. Many won't make any efforts to educate themselves on how to get well, or take the necessary steps they know they should do to help themselves even if their life is at stake. Knowing these aspects of human nature, we are only going to concentrate on the very simplest of supplemental therapies you can use at home that are easy to do without obstacles or supervision.

If you want more extensive alternative protocols, you will need to see a qualified integrative physician or integrative cancer clinic. Only a clinic, physician or other health professional can oversee more complicated therapies that require expert adjustment and monitoring, such as cesium chloride therapy to shrink tumors or hydrazine sulfate therapy.

In other words, if you want more complicated therapies than these then you must consult an experienced cancer expert. You want to deal with qualified experts who know what they are doing. Your life is at stake, and this is not a game of "trial and error." To find those physicians and to find out more details about the many different types of cancer therapies out there, you can read the books already mentioned and also consult experienced cancer coaches who have been dealing with thousands of cancer patients for years. Just a few coaches you might consult include:

- Burton Goldberg at Burtongoldberg.com
- Ralph Moss reports at Cancerdecisions.com
- Bill Henderson at Beating-cancer-gently.com
- Michael Vrentas at Cellectbudwig.com
- Larry at Essense-of-life.com
- Nancy Shaw at TheCancerAlternative.com
- Paul Winter at Alternativecancer.us

In short, your cancer diagnosis doesn't have to be a death sentence. You can use very gentle treatments, such as those within this book, that safely target the destruction of cancer cells or help revert them to normal cells, and which can work by themselves or in conjunction with standard cancer medical therapies. However, to do so you must be willing to cultivate a different mindset than the typical patient who blindly trusts doctors and only does what they are told. When you honestly look at the actual track records of mainstream therapies and see how ineffective they can sometimes be, you will realize you can no longer remain just a passive patient on the mainstream medical conveyor who hopes that traditional cancer treatments by themselves will be enough to help you survive.

You must be willing to fight to save your life, and to fight wisely you must educate yourself on the best treatment options, while also learning how to assist the healing process with supplemental, adjunctive therapies at home. You must remember that if you don't get well then you are going to die, so you must be willing to change your life in a dramatic way to correct what might have produced cancer in the first place. You should be willing to do everything helpful that might assist in your healing process to prevent a terminal outcome.

You must choose to do something extra, especially since the mainstream protocols might be the very things that weaken you to the point of death. There are many supplemental therapies that sometimes produce cures just on their own, and so we will now introduce some of the simplest and easiest of these at home therapies that you might immediately use.

2
CANCER DIET PRINCIPLES

The first step to beating cancer is changing your diet to support your health and healing. Conventional medicine will often tell you that nutrition isn't that important in fighting cancer, or that healthy nutritional protocols can interfere with modern treatments such as chemotherapy and make them less effective. This just isn't true. You need to be healthy to survive and that survival depends on good nutrition. Nutritional and nutraceutical supplements can help you secure this nutrition.

According to information from our national cancer organizations, almost all cancers are caused by diet and environmental factors. The causes of cancer can include smoking, estrogen mimicking chemicals, radiation damage, EMFs, solvents, pesticides, environmental toxins and pollution. We also have such possibilities as viruses and bacteria, heavy metals, GMO foods and trans-fatty acids. Basically, most of the possible causes of cancer are related to our environment, diet and lifestyle. Various studies also show that there is a very high likelihood that your diet has played some role in producing (or not sufficiently preventing) your cancer.

In the presence of these causal factors, the body becomes weakened and cancer cells easily develop like seeds placed in a fertile soil that encourage their growth. Tumors form, which metastasize, and then the cancer becomes a generalized systemic, chronic condition. A tumor is only the outward symptom of the disease, so if you just cut it out or radiate it away, you have not "cured cancer" at all because you haven't addressed the underlying systemic imbalance that caused it. You have not corrected the underlying biochemical terrain. However, diet and supplements can definitely help you do that, which is why they are essential in any medical regimen designed to eliminate cancer.

Even if you insist that diet had nothing to do with your cancer because you have a "genetic predisposition" for immune problems like cancer, those genetic predispositions are usually activated because of what you do or don't eat. Therefore, if you claim you got cancer "due to genetics" then your diet is still probably at fault in some way. If we look at how infrequently cancer used to occur in the past, we can surmise that it has increased in frequency precisely because we have veered too far from healthy habits, with the major contributor being a poor diet.

Since your diet has probably helped you to become sick, your diet can also play a major role in helping you to get well again. It is "rule number one" for cancer patients that you are going to have to clean up your diet to maximize your chances of beating cancer for good.

Changing your diet can certainly help cure you because your diet and nutrition are not secondary concerns, but are actually *the core of any successful cancer treatment*. Your diet can make your internal terrain hostile to cancer cells. It can strengthen and rebuild your immune system. It can actually help your body to target cancer cells for destruction, or supply nutrients that help them revert to normal cells, and it can protect your normal cells while you undergo various cancer treatments that would normally hurt you. At the minimum, the right diet will help you remain strong as your cancer progresses and you undergo any mainstream or other therapies.

Certain anti-cancer diets are so successful that the alternative medicine field considers them cancer treatments by themselves. The truth, however, is that while your diet can be an anti-cancer therapy, *it is usually not strong enough by itself to help you get well*. It is ultra important in helping you get well, but must be considered just a part of a larger overall healing protocol.

From this point forward, you should understand that your diet is just as important as the rest of your treatment protocols, whatever they are. From this point onward, you must understand that your diet will play a major role in whether your cancer spreads or goes into remission.

If you have already beaten cancer, *your diet will also play a significant role in whether you stay well and keep cancer at bay.* Many people use mainstream therapies to send cancer into remission and then, neglecting their diet, see it reappear years later when it could easily have been avoided by sticking to some simple dietary rules. If you are trying to prevent cancer, this certainly means eating many cancer-protective or cancer-killing foods and supplements that activate the genes that protect you from cancer. Please recognize all these facts and after reading this chapter, act accordingly.

When you already have cancer, you must remember that beneficial nutrition will make you feel stronger and more energetic, and will therefore enable you to better handle various orthodox cancer therapies that will put a burden on your body. Nutritional therapy will certainly make you more comfortable and can help you to endure the poisonous troubles of chemotherapy. It can help prevent infections and help you heal better after chemotherapy, surgery or radiation therapy, too. A poor diet, on the other hand, *can undermine any cancer treatments* and may even cancel out their good effects.

Many studies show that nutrition improves the results of chemotherapy, surgery and radiation, while reducing unwanted side effects. In some cases of cancer, special nutritional protocols even do a better job than chemotherapy itself, so it is impossible to say that your diet and nutrition do not matter much when you are fighting cancer. A cancer patient nourished through proper eating and beneficial supplements can definitely secure a better quality of life, longer life and improved chances for a complete cancer remission. It is absolutely wrong to say that nutrition is counterproductive to cancer treatments or that it offsets chemotherapy's effectiveness or the efficacy of other mainstream cancer therapies.

You should also understand that while chemotherapy typically targets a single gene or limited set of genes, a nutritional approach to healing can work on thousands of genes simultaneously, which is what you want to have happening. Cancer specialist Dr. Stanislaw Burzynski has said that an average cancer has about 80 abnormal genes but can have as many as 500; the average number of abnormal genes in a tumor ranges from 40 to 200 yet can even total as much as 2,000. Even so, doctors are still not using combinations of gene-targeted medications in their therapies, or even genetically testing cancers for which medications would be the most effective. A typical cancer medication might target just a few abnormal genes in your tumor, whereas a natural substance like vitamin D has an influence over 2,000 genes in your body, which is why it is so important for cancer prevention.

Nutritional therapy is so powerful because it works on affecting hundreds of genes at the same time. It works on many curative angles and biochemical processes rather than just one. Since many cancer patients die from cachexia or malnutrition, these are yet additional reasons why your nutritional diet and various nutritional supplements should be a top concern at this time.

Your diet can feed the flames of cancer or help to put them out. In short, your diet *may be the most significant factor to defeating cancer*, despite a physician telling you that their medical treatment is of paramount importance. Few cancer treatments will be more effective than changing your diet for the better (since it can feed healthy cells, attack cancerous cells or even starve them to death), and that is the truth regardless of what the medical establishment may sometimes tell you. As you know, because it can change your internal biochemical terrain which is the cause of the problem, some people have even reversed cases of cancer through their diet alone.

How far you go with your anti-cancer diet is up to you, but this much is clear. The right type of diet can play a big role in reversing cancer and helping you stay well. Therefore to get well, you must first correct any dietary factors that played a role in encouraging the growth and development of your cancer. Second, you should not continue feeding cancer through bad dietary habits while working to get rid of it.

In short, now is the time to switch to a more beneficial diet that helps to cure cancer instead of strengthening it. Even if your diet cannot cure cancer, the right type of nutritional support through food and supplements can help protect you against the toxic effects of chemotherapy and radiation (if you choose to use them), without reducing their effectiveness in eliminating cancer at all. They can help you to get stronger so that you have the energy and means to heal.

There are literally dozens of books on the optimum anti-cancer diet that will help you prevent cancer, strengthen your immune system or even lead to a cancer cure. Most of these diets will insist that you *do not eat sugar* because tumors feed on sugar and it also depresses your immune system. They will tell you to avoid foods and substances that cause cancer or internal inflammation. They will tell you to *avoid toxins* that put a burden on your body such as fluoride, chlorine, or food additives and chemicals (such as aspartame, saccharin, sulphites, MSG, nitrates and nitrites). They will tell you to *avoid allergenic foods and food sensitivities* that put an extra burden on your immune system when it is already taxed to the fullest. They will tell you to eat foods that support your eliminatory organs and the detoxification systems of your body, such as your liver and kidneys.

Many diets will also tell you to especially *avoid GMO foods* since GMO foods consistently cause cancer tumors or organ failure in animals, especially in the liver and kidneys. If you don't believe that GMO foods can cause tumors, organ failure, gastric lesions, liver damage, kidney damage, allergic reactions and organ dysfunction, you have been hoodwinked by the public relations campaigns of the GMO industry and need to educate yourself quickly, because your life is on the line when you continue to eat these foods. I will make it simple for you: as various researchers are showing, GMO foods can and do cause cancer, and nutritionists and physicians definitively report that a wide variety of health conditions improve after people switch back to eating non-GMO foods.

If you are still eating GMO foods (such as GMO corn and soy) while trying to get rid of cancer, chances are that your cancer will not go away or is likely to return even if you do eliminate it. In addition to causing infertility, organ failure, organ dysfunction and tumors, GMO products are also usually allergenic foods that cause the unwanted immunological response of inflammation. Since you want to remove all allergenic foods from your diet when fighting cancer, this is another reason to completely remove GMO foods from your diet even if you don't think they are cancer causing. Basically, you should eliminate GMO foods from your diet. You will find that eliminating harmful food offenders from your diet will probably have a bigger effect than adding beneficial foods, and this especially applies to eliminating GMO substances from consumption.

When we look at all this information, the basic principles of an anti-cancer diet are that there are *foods you should avoid and foods you should eat*. You want to avoid anything that may potentially cause cancer or feed it, thus helping it to spread. You want to eat foods that attack cancer and thwart it from spreading, or which change your internal terrain to make it more difficult for cancer to survive and grow. You also want to use aggressive nutritional protocols to supply yourself with nutrients that bolster your normal healthy cells, correct internal imbalances and support your immune system in its task of eradicating cancer.

VARIOUS CANCER DIETS

Many diets have therefore been proposed for eliminating cancer. As just a few examples there is the macrobiotic diet (*The Cancer Prevention Diet*, *The Macrobiotic Approach to Cancer*), ketogenic diet, raw food diet (*Eating in the Raw*, *Maximize Immunity*), Hallelujah Acres diet, Dries cancer diet (*The Dries Cancer Diet*), alkaline diet (*Eating the Alkaline Way* or *Preventive Medical Research* by Dr. Bernardo Majalca), Breuss Diet (*The Breuss Cancer Cure*), Budwig diet (*A Day in the Budwig Diet*), Brandt Grape Cure diet (*The Grape Cure*), Robert Young pH diet (*Sick and Tired? – Reclaim Your Inner Terrain*), Moerman diet (*Dr. Moerman's Anti-cancer Diet*), Johannes Kuhl lactic-acid-fermented foods diet, and raw juicing diets such as the Gerson diet (*The Gerson Therapy*, *Healing the Gerson Way*).

There are so many anti-cancer diets that it is hard to choose one. However, while they embody various different approaches to help you beat cancer, they usually rely on some common principles such as avoiding sugar, white flour products and processed foods, eating clean foods, avoiding GMO products, alkalizing the body and so on.

If you are fighting cancer, it makes sense that you need to find the right diet *for you*. This should be an individualized determination rather than a one-size-fits-all decision. "One cancer diet for everyone" does not make sense because different physiologies and pathologies may need different approaches to beating cancer. Even the supplements you may take to help yourself should greatly depend upon your dietary patterns and physical circumstances.

For instance, famous alternative cancer therapist William Donald Kelley (who treated over 33,000 patients) is said to have achieved a 93% cure rate with newly diagnosed cancers using entirely different anti-cancer diets for different body types, and he designed his highly successful protocols around this idea. He had different diets for patients ranging from 100% vegetarian nut and seed diets to those requiring that patients eat red meat three times per day. Dr. Nicholas Gonzalez, who has expanded on Kelley's work, now uses ninety different variations that are based on each of the ten basic diets!

Every individual is different, and when the problem of compliance is added in we therefore cannot say that there is one best cancer fighting diet for everyone. For instance, some diets are just "too foreign" for certain blood types or meat eaters to handle, and the difficulty of adapting means they usually won't be followed. Therefore there is *no one perfect diet* for everyone when we are fighting cancer because compliance must be taken into account. There are many possible different dietary approaches, and your own anti-cancer diet must be selected according to your situation, including your ability to follow it. It may also change dramatically depending upon whether you are an early stage or late stage cancer patient.

In short, the best anti-cancer diet *for you* depends upon your situation, and you should decide upon this diet after sitting down and discussing matters with a qualified health practitioner who is skilled in these matters. You need to talk to an expert about this important decision and it must take into consideration whether or not you will actually follow the diet proposed.

If you don't factor the likelihood of compliance into consideration, you might determine there is an "optimum" diet just right for your condition, but that dietary strategy will be useless because you don't like it and won't stick with it. As many doctors will lament, some people absolutely will not change any harmful dietary patterns or lifestyles even though faced with impending death. Therefore, since some patients may be able to follow something "less optimal" to the letter while they could not follow what is "best," this is something you should factor into the diet selection process. The "best diet" is not necessarily the ultimate, best diet for your body. In short, the best diet for you may be a diet that is beneficial for your health, but also a diet which you are able to follow on a consistent basis.

The Gerson diet, as an example, is a famous cancer curative diet that requires a great deal of commitment that many people just don't have. The Gerson diet is essentially a strict vegetarian, fat-free and salt-free diet that requires that you drink great quantities of fresh vegetable juice. You must also avoid all dairy, soy and fried foods. The diet is demanding and will consume much of your day just in preparation alone. All day long you are drinking fresh vegetable juice, which helps detoxify your body while placing a lower energy burden on your digestive system. How many people have the time and discipline to follow this on their own unless they are at a clinic?

All of the principles within the Gerson diet are extremely important. Its rules are designed to eliminate the underlying causes of most diseases, so as to produce lasting cures for a large number of degenerative health conditions. However, the diet is so restrictive that it is difficult for many people to follow, and if they veer from the diet then it usually results in failure. The same is said of the macrobiotic diet in that you must be extremely committed to the diet to be able to follow its many restrictions and maintain it. If you cannot do that, wouldn't it be better to face the truth and devote yourself to following a less optimal yet still beneficial anti-cancer diet, namely one that you can maintain?

You must think carefully about these things because this frank discussion alone might be the one thing that saves your life. It might help you decide to remain compliant with a diet that is strict rather than simply eat whatever you want and then die due to a lack of discipline. As stated, many of the alternative, integrative therapies may not be able to cure cancer, *but they may be able to help you reach a point where you can manage it as an ongoing chronic condition, like diabetes,* if you have the right discipline. The diet plays a major role in this strategy.

In any case, all cancer patients need to be aware of some basic dietary principles that feed cancer, some that thwart cancer, and some that lead to healing in general because they boost your immune system, reduce inflammation, detoxify a lifetime accumulation of toxins and help you repair your DNA. You should remember these dietary principles regardless of whatever diet you choose to follow. Just knowing these principles will usually help you decide whether to put a fork in your mouth which contains food that may affect your health, so we will discuss them.

Focusing on principles in this way, rather than advocating that you follow a certain specific diet, will serve you better in helping you to find an anti-cancer diet that you can follow. Once again, after you understand these principles you can more intelligently discuss the issue with a qualified health professional to help determine which diet is *best for you*.

You should also certainly buy the books specific to that diet, such as the ones previously mentioned, so that you can easily learn how to follow it. This is not a book focused on cancer diets, however, so all we can do is give you some basic information to help you get started at cleaning up your diet immediately, and which is applicable regardless of what final diet you select.

For all cancer diets, basically there are some foods you should eat and some you should avoid because they would work against the objective of eliminating cancer. Therefore, if you incorporate the following principles into your diet, you will be taking steps in the right direction by nutritionally supporting your body to get well:

1. You must stop eating foods that cancer cells love, and most of all they love sugar (glucose) because their metabolism uses it to grow. *Our bodies easily turn sugar into glucose, which actually feeds cancer*, so you must remove sugar from your diet as much as possible to stop feeding it. This is the main dietary therapy for treating cancer, which is to starve it of its food source by denying it any easy glucose. Cancer cells typically use eight times more glucose than normal cells, thriving on glucose because they cannot metabolize complex carbohydrates, so you should remove all simple sugars as much as possible from your diet to deny fueling cancer with what it needs for survival. Since eating sugar also temporarily *depresses your immune system for several hours*, this is another reason to remove it from your diet. While vitamin C typically "wakes up" your immune system, one "dose" of sugar can depress your immune system and thus temporarily reduce your ability to fight cancer. Sugar also *feeds any fungus and yeast in your body*, which increases the total burden on your immune system when your body is busy trying to fight cancer. All these reasons tell us that you absolutely MUST reduce your sugar intake. Avoid all forms of sugar in your diet, including sucrose and high-fructose corn syrup. You should also eliminate

grain-based foods and foods with a high glycemic index (wheat flour products, white rice, white potatoes, white bread, white pastas, corn, etc.) that metabolize into glucose quickly within the body. This includes the refined grains, namely wheat flour products such as pancakes, donuts, bread, pasta, pastries, desserts and so on. It additionally includes alcohol, soda pop, milk and dairy products unless we are talking about dairy products specifically used for a particular anti-cancer diet therapy (such as the cottage cheese used for the Budwig mixture). The basic principle is to eliminate all sorts of refined sugars and refined carbohydrates from your diet. Sugar feeds nearly every chronic disease but it especially fuels cancer cells and keeps them alive, so you must stop eating it as much as possible. It is as simple as that. You must avoid all forms of sugar because they feed cancer directly or support microbes in your body that overburden your immune system when you want it to be in tiptop condition fighting cancer.

2. You must remove from your diet *any foods that are known to cause cancer*. This includes "trans fats" that are produced during the frying process (and also in margarine), MSG, nitrate and nitrite (found in processed meats such as hot dogs, bacon, salami, etc.) and man-made sweeteners such as aspartame, NutraSweet and Equal as well as the products which contain them (such as most diet sodas). One of the biggest cancer-causing food categories is GMO foods, which animal studies definitely prove are cancer-causing or tied to allergies, infertility and organ failure. They are also often treated with heavy doses of herbicides or pesticides that are likely to be carcinogenic. You absolutely MUST remove all GMO foods from your diet if you want to permanently beat cancer, otherwise it is likely to come back when it seems to be gone. GMO foods definitely can cause tumors and organ failure! Since the major GMO crops are **soybeans and corn**, which are allergens for many people anyway, they should be removed from your diet to follow the principle of no longer suppressing your immune system in any way. Soy products, when unfermented, should also be avoided for other reasons as well. A whole book could be written on the dangers of eating unfermented soy products, but this is a lengthy topic you might investigate for yourself.

3. You should eliminate *any food allergies, sensitivities or intolerances* from your diet because, as noted, they will produce internal inflammation that puts further stress on your immune system, thus distracting it from fighting cancer. To determine your allergies, food sensitivities and intolerances, you should get tested by a qualified physician. Eight foods typically produce the most negative reactions: soy, peanuts, corn, eggs, sugar, gluten (mainly wheat), dairy, and GMO. As you can see, many of the same foods are appearing on multiple "do not eat" lists, so they should be avoided for multiple reasons. Some people are also allergic to the nightshade vegetables (tomatoes, potatoes, chili peppers, eggplant, tobacco and paprika), so these may or may not be problematical. Basically, eating the wrong foods can damage your body or weaken your immune system. However, if you *remove your dietary sources of immune stress and inflammation*, you might find that subtracting harmful foods from your diet has a bigger effect on treating a health condition than adding beneficial ones. As you are probably realizing, all these injunctions are just common sense principles but unfortunately not common knowledge held by the general public.

4. Eliminate foods that *feed yeast and fungus* within your body, or foods where yeast, fungus or mold is present. Peanuts, which are often covered with fungus, are an example of such a food to avoid (and it is a common allergen, too). As mentioned, sugar feeds yeast within your body, as do the grains, so the "white foods" that previously appeared on "avoid lists" have yet another reason to be avoided once again. The purpose of eliminating these foods from your diet is to help create an internal immunological terrain that is better able to resist and fight cancer. A caveat: just as we saw that dairy is permitted when it is used in a specific cancer therapy, some mushroom products (ex. such as those containing beta 1,3D glucans) are used in immune-stimulating cancer protocols and thus permitted even though they are fungi. When foods are used in specific alternative treatment protocols, such as honey though sugar should usually be avoided, there is a reason you can make an exception from the general principle.

5.   You need to eliminate any foods, ingredients or chemicals that interfere with alternative and mainstream treatments for cancer, such as chlorine and fluoride (which cause cancer), alcohol and coffee. If you develop cancer, you definitely need to drink clean water (such as spring water) and wash with clean water, so if you can afford to, immediately get a quality water filter and shower filter for your home because your body absorbs some of these chemicals through the skin. Consider a reverse osmosis water filter for your drinking water, but remember that this single act isn't going to save you, so *put your time and energy into other therapies most of all.* If you have your home checked and find out that EMFs are a problem, you can eliminate them as a source of trouble by using some of the devices at TooMuchEmf.com. You should avoid wearing makeup, or instead can switch to natural beauty products. You will often feel better from just this small change alone. Most cosmetics contain estrogen-mimicking compounds that cause cancer and surprisingly, a woman's body usually absorbs up to two pounds of cosmetics per year through the skin.

6.   Some anti-cancer diets include meats, while some are entirely vegetarian because animal proteins often feed cancer. Nonetheless, while meats are acid-producing foods and can contribute to getting cancer, you don't have to be afraid of eating animal protein. You must consume enough protein to build healthy cells when you get cancer, which is a fact that many vegetarian cancer diets neglect. The major principle is to switch to *eating clean foods* which means that if you are a meat eater, you should turn to organic free range and grass fed meats – preferably organic meats and eggs – and try to avoid frying or charbroiling them. You don't necessarily need to be vegetarian to fight cancer even though it is true that most anti-cancer diets have a vegetarian emphasis. There are raw food diets that have successfully cured countless diseases, and vegetable juicing diets, too, which you might consider if you know how to supply yourself with enough protein. While sugar should be avoided in most anti-cancer diets, the sugars in cancer-killing fruits and vegetables (such as carrots or blueberries) are permitted in these juicing protocols. Carrot juice, for instance, is not a problem. If you want to juice, you should

read some books containing the many vegetable juicing do's and don'ts for fighting cancer, such as taught with the Gerson diet. Most raw vegetable juices should be produced by from organic vegetables having known cancer-fighting abilities such as carrots, broccoli, cauliflower, cabbage, asparagus, and red beets. The fruits having known cancer-fighting abilities include purple grapes (with skins and seeds), blueberries, raw pineapple, red and black raspberries, strawberries, peaches and apricots, mangosteen, noni, wolfberry and goji berries. Wheatgrass and barley grass juice, by themselves, are also often considered highly beneficial for curing cancer. For instance, wheatgrass contains many anti-cancer agents such as chlorophyll, selenium, laetrile and abscisic acid, and is one of the most alkaline-producing foods known. Any green superfoods are recommended because they typically contain the concentrated juice powders (that are easily digested and absorbed) of all sorts of anti-cancer botanicals. Good nutritional balance is needed when fighting cancer, and many of the concentrated green superfood powders fit this bill. They will especially help patients to better deal with chemotherapy should they choose it.

If you embark upon a road of better nutrition from following simple dietary principles like this, this will make you feel stronger, give you more energy, help you heal faster and make you more comfortable for any cancer condition. These rules can even help to protect you against the side effects of toxic chemotherapy. A better diet is hugely important because this is what *establishes the necessary solid foundation* for all the cancer treatments you choose to undertake. A good diet will help your body win the war against cancer, and then help to keep cancer away for good.

When you examine all these dietary principles, the basic idea they communicate is that you want to stay away from eating junk food. You want to clean up your diet by eating "clean, high quality" foods to replace all the processed junk food you normally consume. Instead of eating nutrient-depleted junk food, you want to replace it with real nourishment. It is paramount to clean up your diet in this way because you won't be able to rebuild your health if your nutrition is off and you are not supplying your ailing body with the right materials so that it can build healthy new cells.

If you are a meat eater, "clean, high quality" food means consuming free range, grass fed, organic meat. Less meat in the diet is also usually better than more, and the diet should be tipped toward the side of more organic fruits and vegetables. Since we are talking about greens, this means eating pesticide-free, *organic* vegetables and fruits. Basically, you must also replace chemical-laden processed food with fresh wholesome foods instead. Furthermore, you should avoid the unhealthy fats and oils that weaken your body's cell membranes (making them susceptible to cancer) and excess alcohol consumption.

Some anti-cancer diets insist that you should eat raw food, which works for some individuals, but in all cases it should certainly be ripe, fresh, organic and free of chemicals. If we are talking about cooked food, remember that many cancer doctors will recommend that you take digestive enzymes with your meals. This is especially important if chemotherapy ends up destroying your digestive system, as it commonly does. Some cancer diets recommend the juicing of fresh fruits and vegetables, which will add many highly absorbable forms of vitamins and minerals to your diet, but the particular juicing routines proposed will depend upon the specific diet plan being recommended.

There are countless cancer-protective foods and cancer-killing fruits and vegetables, and you should certainly try to include them in your diet. Why would you want to avoid them? When undergoing chemotherapy, you must ask yourself, "Chemotherapy is creating toxicity, so how can I protect my health and get stronger so that I can better deal with it?" Even if you aren't undergoing chemotherapy or radiation, you still have to think, "What should I eat that will help me to reverse my cancer?"

Some of the foods which contain powerful nutrients that kill cancer cells, stop the spread of cancer, or address the problem of cancer in some other way include curcumin (found in turmeric), paprika, broccoli, cauliflower, Brussel sprouts, kale, cabbage, carrots, almonds, red raspberries, black raspberries, strawberries and purple grapes. These foods contain helpful nutritional substances like carotenoids, lycopene, sulforaphane, flavonoids, zeaxanthin or indole-3-carbonale. Purple grapes, for instance, contain over a dozen cancer-killing nutrients.

Using the internet you can readily find lists of foods you should avoid and foods you should eat for any health condition. You can also readily find cancer food lists. However, what is more important than a list of foods are the dietary principles we have covered, as well as the various supplemental therapies that can help send cancer into remission.

ANTI-CANCER SUPPLEMENTS AND NUTRACEUTICALS

In terms of additional dietary things you can do to help yourself, there are literally hundreds of foods and supplements to choose from when fighting cancer and the vast number of choices can be overwhelming, especially when you have just learned you have cancer and you are now in a rush, trying to find out how you can help yourself as quickly as possible.

You absolutely cannot consume everything said to be good for you (some of which can even work against other therapies you might be using), nor could you afford this approach! Sometimes, however, you just have to do something that will immediately start buying you more time so that various other cancer treatment therapies have a chance to help you get well. But what are the fewest but most powerful things you can do that won't interfere with anything that doctors would normally do for you?

While cost may or may not be a consideration, you certainly need some way to beneficially prioritize the many possibilities to choose from. In terms of nutritional supplements, it comes down to intelligently determining which ones are likely to bring you the biggest benefits possible for your condition.

One of the best information sources on helpful anti-cancer supplements comes from Patrick Quillan, author of *Beating Cancer With Nutrition*. Quillan once offered an excellent nutritional powder, called Immunopower, which contained an extensive number of ingredients known to fight against cancer, so that you didn't have to shop for individual supplements on your own. While it solved the problem of being easy to consume and was one of the best values for money available anywhere for a comparable regimen (75% cheaper than buying all the necessary supplements individually), he had to take it off the market because it was still too expensive for most patients.

For an excellent green powder supplement today you will now have to turn to other products filled with beneficial ingredients such as Boku Superfood, Vitamineral Green, Pure Synergy, SuperGreens (InnerLight), ProGreens or some other supergreens formula. If you carefully examine the ingredients of these various products, you may start to suspect that some were especially formulated with the idea of fighting cancer in mind, but the companies cannot market their products this way. Concentrated food products known to help with cancer, such as green barley grass or wheatgrass juice, are also readily available for purchase as well.

Because of their rich nutrient content, many of these powders can help protect your body or keep a cancer sufferer alive long enough so that they have more time to attack their cancer with other effective therapies. Some may also help participate in producing a cancer cure by boosting your immune system or supplying nutrients that attack cancer directly. You can also combine several of these powders together because you want to include the ingredients that are the most important. For instance, sometimes protecting the stomach and intestines from the bad effects of chemotherapy ("chemotherapy induced gastrointestinal damage") is as simple as adding 4 grams of glutamine powder to a scoop of one of these green powders and consuming this twice a day on a consistent basis. While this is extremely important to know, it is information that your doctor is unlikely to tell you.

Cellect, which is another special nutritional product you should consider, is a nutritional powder developed by the president of the National Cancer Research Foundation (Fred Eichorn), and has shown excellent results with many forms of cancer (see Cellect.org). In addition to Cellect, there are also specific anti-cancer foods/supplements that contain many ingredients such as Oncolyn and LifeOne. However, these are anti-cancer supplements you should use under the guidance of an expert. Since cancer is the result of an accumulation of imbalances and toxicities, an expert will usually need to help determine which of these products/approaches can be most beneficial to your condition.

The difficulty of picking the right nutritional supplements to fight cancer that you can use on your own without much supervision, and the fact that they can be expensive, is why this book concentrates on the fewest relatively inexpensive things that have the greatest chance to do the most good. At this point in time, you don't want to have to consider hundreds of possible supplements. As stated, you could neither afford them all or take them. You need to concentrate on absorbing information that permits action to follow rather than try to learn about many different supplements and cancer theories that would be of no use to you. You should immediately focus on the fewest powerful things you can do/take that might be complements to traditional cancer therapies and which might also be considered treatments by themselves.

Once again, picking the right supplements to help fight your cancer is an individual decision that must be made dependent upon your condition. As an example, famous cancer therapist Dr. William Kelley felt that vegetarians did well with potassium, magnesium, vitamin C and B-vitamin supplements but not with vitamin E. He felt that meat eaters did well with calcium, zinc, selenium and vitamin E supplements, but did poorly with magnesium and potassium. In other words, some people will do phenomenally well on a particular diet, while others will crash on that same diet plan. Along the same principle, there are few supplements that are right for everyone, so to determine the best supplements to take it is best to talk to an expert.

Even with this variety, there are some standard common principles to cancer supplementation that should be kept in mind. Some supplements can help you with energy, pain or suffering. Some will help your body with the burden of detoxifying the results of cancer treatments, since they start to destroy cells within your body. Some will attack cancer cells directly or help them revert back to normal, thus helping other therapies to become more effective or serving as standalone therapies. Some will help to rebuild your immune system, and so on.

There are several basic supplements you should know about that are usually included within many integrative cancer protocols. You should know about these options because they usually can serve as safe adjunctive additions to most mainstream cancer treatment protocols:

- **Cold pressed organic flaxseed oil and cottage cheese**. Fresh flaxseed oil is used in many cancer curative protocols, such as the **Budwig diet**, and a special cottage cheese and flaxseed oil combination should be added to your diet. In the 1950s, German biochemist Dr. Joanna

Budwig extensively studied the blood of cancer patients and from her extensive research, she hypothesized that a dietary deficiency of the right type of electron-rich fatty acids induced the growth of cancer cells. Her book, *Cancer – The Problem and the Solution*, was written after fifty years of successfully treating cancer patients with what was said to be a nearly 90% cure rate if her protocols were started early enough and followed correctly. Her dietary formulas, using the unsaturated fats provided by flaxseed oil, give the body special omega-3 fatty acids that build stronger cell membranes and transfer more oxygen into cancer cells so that the body returns to normal. The idea is that flaxseed oil helps to correct a particular dietary fatty acid deficiency that then allows weak cell membranes to repair themselves, which is an entirely different approach to cancer than that the poison-based attack of chemotherapy. The most famous Budwig dietary protocol involves mixing four tablespoons of low-fat organic cottage cheese with two tablespoons of fresh flaxseed oil to supply the appropriate electron-rich fatty acids to the body. Cancer patients should slowly work up to consuming 4-8 tablespoons of flaxseed oil per day in this mixture, and must consume the cottage cheese/flaxseed oil mixture *immediately* after it is made. This food quickly negates the damaging effects of cancer cells and helps protect healthy cells by adjusting the electrical charge in and around those cells. There are many thousands of documented cases of cancer remissions from individuals who have used the Budwig diet and who credit Dr. Budwig for their life, but it usually takes 3-6 months to see results. Furthermore, it helps only with certain types of cancers, usually those less advanced and those with solid mass tumors rather than systemic cancers, such as lymphomas, or cancers metastasized to the bone. In any case, to make her famous flaxseed oil mixture, you can use Barleans and other flaxseed oil brands that are readily available in health food stores or on the internet. The main requirement is that the flaxseed oil be organic, cold-pressed and unrefined. Salad oils, mayonnaise, margarine, butter, animal fats and fried foods should also be avoided because they supply the body with "bad fats" rather than the good fatty aids needed by cancer cells to repair themselves. Cottage cheese is part of the Budwig mixture because it contains sulfurated (sulfur-containing) proteins help the body to use the fatty acids of the flaxseed oil more efficiently. It makes them water soluble so that they can pass easily through the body and readily become bio-available to cells. Studies on cancer using the flaxseed oil alone without sulfurated proteins do not show anything near the anti-cancer results that Budwig achieved. Is this Joanna Budwig cottage cheese-flaxseed oil mixture in any way contraindicated by mainstream cancer treatments? No! It's just a food that lowers inflammation, helps your body to repair old cells and build healthy new cellular membranes, helps detoxify the body and also happens to revert cancer cells quite nicely. You can readily pick up several books on the Budwig diet to see how to incorporate it into your life. However, in particular you should read Bill Henderson's books, *Beating Cancer Gently* and *Cancer-Free,* to learn how to incorporate the Budwig "flaxseed oil and cottage cheese" protocol into a larger set of very effective natural cancer therapies which you can easily use on your own. All cancer patients should consider adding the cottage cheese-flaxseed oil mixture to their diet.

- **Selenium,** like iodine, calcium, magnesium, zinc, vitamin D and vitamin C, has been proven to be essential in helping to beat cancer. It is a key mineral involved in both cancer prevention and many alternative cancer treatment protocols because it inhibits metastasis. Many famous doctors who have achieved extremely high cancer cure rates, such as Dr. Emanuel Revici (see *The Doctor Who Cures Cancer* by William Eidem), have used very high dosages of selenium in curative protocols because, like platinum, it helps prevent damaged DNA from proliferating during mitosis, thus preventing tumors from developing. It also helps kill cancer cells, too. To use selenium effectively, Revici developed unique lipid envelopes for selenium molecules so that he could safely deliver intravenous dosages as high as 10 grams to a patient. These high dosages would only dissolve once inside of cancer cells, thus destroying tumors from the inside out. Selenium therefore works similarly to laetrile and other special botanicals by destroying cancer cells from the inside after it is absorbed. You definitely should add some degree of selenium to your diet when you have cancer, so the question is which selenium supplement is best. The typical choices include sodium selenite, selenomethionine, or methylselenocysteine supplements, but the best option is probably "**Phytosel,**" which is a natural selenium tablet derived from hydroponically grown mustard greens. This is selenium derived from a plant-based source. It can be taken at high doses without side effects and is readily available from Ojibwa Tea of Life (Ojibwatea.com 303-322-7930). You can find more about selenium's use for cancer in various publications, such as John Boik's *Natural Compounds in Cancer Therapy* and Mark Konlee's *Immune Restoration Handbook*. Nearly every cancer book will discuss and recommend the use of selenium, which is much more effective when there is a high level of vitamin E in the blood (the A.C. Grace "Ultimate E" brand is recommended). Consult an expert for the recommended preventive dosage (200-400 mcg/day) or therapeutic dosage (900-2000 mcg/day) within a comprehensive cancer regimen.

- **Mineral supplements** - Trace minerals (elements), which are essential for all the body's biochemical processes, are often no longer found in our intensively farmed and depleted agricultural soils, so nearly everyone is nutritionally deficient of these in their diet. You must be getting enough of these trace minerals through your diet, otherwise you should take them through dietary supplements or you will often become unhealthy. Some theories suggest that cancer starts because of nutritional deficiencies like this that affect many of the body's vital processes, and very importantly the body's pH balance. For instance, Fred Eichorn of the National Cancer Research Foundation believes that uncorrected nutritional deficiencies lead to the activation of DNA instructions for alternate ways to produce hormones and amino acids, and these changes may lead to cancer. Regardless as to whether this is true or not, it is commonly known that you need trace minerals for many biochemical processes. Correcting various trace mineral deficiencies will therefore help to correct any "out of balance" internal biochemistry conditions that are contributing to the development of cancer. While there are good reasons for taking selective forms of selenium, iodine, calcium, sulfur, silver, zinc, cesium and other minerals as curative aids when you have cancer, a general-purpose trace mineral supplement is also of interest in order to supply whatever might help your body to heal. People who take trace minerals commonly report remarkable improvements in their health for all sorts of conditions. **Trace Minerals Research** is one company that offers a highly absorbable form of trace minerals, as does **Goldstake Minerals**, which offers highly absorbable oxide and hydroxide forms of trace minerals mined from an ancient seabed of dioxide clay in Nevada. Originally used by native Americans, they have been used for cancer treatment and many other illnesses since the 1970s, with people reporting tremendous improvements in their health. They are readily available at GoldstakeMinerals.net (800-523-4653). To help re-mineralize a body suffering from deficiencies, a common dosage is 4-6 capsules/day, whereas cancer patients usually take 8-12 capsules/day.

- **Enzymes** – Physicians recommend that cancer patients use enzymes in different ways. For instance, chemotherapy kills or damages fast-growing cells, which are found in your immune system, stomach lining and colon. This harms your ability to digest food. When your stomach or colon is damaged, any nutritional protocol will thereafter never be enough to help you beat cancer because you won't be able to properly digest your foods and supplements. You may therefore want to take digestive enzymes with meals to help your digestion, using popular brands such as "**AbsorbAid**" by Nature's Sources. To get rid of Candida, yeast and fungus to help unburden your immune system, one of the best enzyme supplements for this purpose is "**Candisol**." You might also want to use a brand of general-purpose enzyme supplements on an empty stomach, such as "**Vitalzym**," to help "eat up" or "digest" debris floating in the blood stream, such as cancer cell remains. Other enzyme brands often used by cancer patients for this purpose include "**Univase Forte**," "**Megazyme Forte**" and "**10Zymes**." Most people who are familiar with Dr. Kelley's pancreatic proteolytic enzymes cancer therapy (Kelleymetabolic.com) know that he used enzymes in yet another way, which was to damage cancer cells so that they might be more easily destroyed. Cancer cells have a sticky mucus/protein coating that may be fifteen times thicker than the fibrin surrounding normal cells. This coating renders them invisible to white blood cells, which therefore cannot destroy them because they aren't recognized. Their thick coating basically makes them immune to attack from natural killer cells. Pancreatic proteolytic enzymes, however, strip away the thick outer protective coating of cancer cells, "de-cloaking" them so that they become susceptible to the body's defenses. This has been one of the most popular European approaches to killing cancer for decades and it even *helps chemotherapy*, since the enzymes will improve the ability of toxic chemicals to enter into cancer cells. Taking pancreatic proteolytic enzymes breaks down circulating complexes in the blood, which helps when there is such an overwhelming number of dying cancer cells in the bloodstream that the immune system has a hard time finding the tumors. The enzymes will also help clear away any debris so that living cancer cells become more visible and the immune system can then focus on destroying them. Proteolytic enzymes will also help to reduce internal inflammation, break up blood cell clumps and thin the blood. They can help counter the adverse side effects of chemotherapy and radiation treatments in many ways, and usually improve the response rates to these therapies. *All cancer patients should therefore consider taking enzymes as part of their overall cancer therapy.* Our body has a limited number of proteolytic enzymes available, since they are preoccupied with the duties of digestion, so there are not enough extra enzymes available to go around fighting cancer. However, if you rearrange your diet so that high protein meals occur during breakfast and lunch only, pancreatic enzymes will then be used to digest food protein for about six hours only. This leaves eighteen hours for the production of pancreatic enzymes to digest cancer cells. Kelley proteolytic enzymes therapy requires that the body be saturated with pancreatic proteolytic enzymes all the time that will then work to dissolve the cancer cells. If cancer cells are weakened, they will then become porous and visible to the immune system, thus other therapies attacking them will become far more effective. Dr. Nicholas Gonzalez (Dr-gonzalez.com), who studied with Dr. Kelley, has performed extensive pancreatic enzyme research and created his own distinctive brand of powerful enzymes. These proteolytic enzymes are available through the Allergy Research/Nutricology brand in a product called "**Pancreas Pork Natural Glandular.**" Most Gonzalez patients take between 90-110 enzyme capsules daily, spread throughout the day. You can learn more about these enzymes in an interview he did with Dr. Joseph Mercola, readily available on the web. Lastly, the ingredients within barley and wheatgrass juice (or powder) also make them broad-spectrum enzyme supplements, but neither are blood thinners since they do not have high levels of proteolytic enzymes. They can be added via green powder formulations to any anti-cancer diet. Every cancer patient should consider using an enzyme protocol with their other mainstream or integrative protocols.

- **Ellagic acid** – Ellagic acid is a natural nutrient typically found in berries of all types, in particular red and black raspberries, blackberries, blueberries, walnuts and other fruits such as pomegranates. It is not a cancer cure but is often added to cancer patient diets because it has been definitively proven to kill several cancer cell lines. Conventional cancer treatments usually kill all cells indiscriminately but ellagic acid *only attacks cancer cells*. It leaves healthy cells alone. In addition to inducing natural cell death for cancer cells, ellagic acid also prevents certain types of cell damage by carcinogens and slows tumor growth. Overall this natural ingredient is considered a strong cancer inhibitor that can kill cancer cells without affecting healthy cells, stop or suppress the development and growth of tumors, and has the ability to inhibit mutations in a cell's DNA. On top of this, ellagic acid also has powerful anti-bacterial and anti-viral properties. Various suppliers and products can be found on the internet, such as **RaspberryGold.com** or "**Ellagic Defense**" by Pure Prescriptions. This is one of the products that is easily combined with green powders containing barley grass, wheatgrass juice, carrot juice, broccoli juice, etc. that you should consider adding to every anti-cancer diet.

- **Immune Builders** – For newly diagnosed cancer patients, boosting the immune system is very important because the presence of cancer tells you that there is a major problem that requires adjustment. However, for advanced cases of cancer you must *primarily focus on nourishing your body's healthy cells to stay alive, rather than concentrate on boosting your immune system*, because there is often not enough time to rebuild your immune system so that it can fight cancer effectively. On the other hand, when early stage cancer patients start undergoing chemotherapy and radiation treatments, these therapies will usually start destroying the body's immune system. Thus, cancer patients should immediately start using immune building protocols to help mitigate these effects. They should also use them during remission to help keep cancer at bay. While you can take many different immune boosting supplements, hoping to supercharge your immune system with nutrients so that it can then better deal with the cancer, this is actually a slow approach that rarely works all by itself. It should only be considered as a supplemental approach used *in addition to* other therapies. Nevertheless, there are many individual substances that can help boost the immune system in some way, such as aloe extracts, aged garlic extract, IP6, MGN-3, AHCC, ABM mushroom (*agaricus blazei murill*), maitaike and shiitake mushrooms, cordyceps, *Phellinus linteus*, beta 1,3D glucans, kombucha, Epicor, BioPro thymic protein, hyperimmunized egg powder, olive leaf extract, Cat's claw, Pau d'arco, colostrum, lactoferrin, vitamin A, and so on. Many such helpful ingredients can be found in powerful immune-stimulating formulations such as Madre Labs **"Immune Punch,"** or in supplements such as Garden of Life **"RM-10 Immune System Food,"** which blends ten immune-stimulating mushrooms. If just a single immune-boosting supplement is desired, **"4Life Transfer Factor Plus"** is considered one of the best immune products available as it has been well studied and proven to be able to increase natural killer cell activity more than 400%. Building and boosting the immune system is important for many reasons, including the fact that some theories of cancer's origins propose that it is actually caused by pathogenic microbes. For instance, the HPV (Human Papillomaviruses) group of viruses is thought to be responsible for many types of cancers, while the CDC stated that the simian SV40 polyomavirus that had contaminated polio vaccines was cancer causing, too. MD Anderson Cancer Center reports that viral agents play a critical role in 20% of reported cancers. According to one version of the cancer-microbe theory, killing pathogenic cancer-causing microbes works better than trying to destroy cancer cells directly because the result is often that cells revert back to normal and thus there is little debris from cancer cells dying. So boosting your immune system to fight viruses and other microbial invaders is also a key factor against these types of cancer. If you can help your body to get rid of these pathogens quickly, you will deny them the time required to produce cancer and will thus help to prevent cancer from developing and spreading. This immunological approach is another entirely different approach than what is typically used in mainstream cancer medicine, and usually safely *complements any mainstream treatment protocols of chemotherapy, surgery or radiation*. Along this line of approach, various other integrative protocols are also available that are designed to carry specially selected immune products into cancer cells to help kill microbes and/or help the cancer cells revert back to normal. Examples are intravenous vitamin C and MSM/DMSO (organic sulfur), etc. As supplemental treatments, various immune products can usually be safely added to the diet and do not normally contradict any traditional cancer therapies.

That's it for a brief introduction to the most common anti-cancer diet principles to know about along with some of the most important nutraceutical supplements to consider, so let us summarize this topic to make it simple.

Many doctors will tell you that nutrition isn't that important in curing cancer, or that it will hurt the outcomes of chemotherapy or radiation. They will tell you to avoid vitamins and supplements during cancer treatments even though you are supposed to continue getting these nutritional ingredients from your food anyway. To say that nutrition is unimportant or that most nutritional supplements are contraindicated by cancer therapies is just plain wrong, as you probably now realize and as many scientific studies clearly prove. Mainstream cancer advice commonly ignores hundreds of research studies that prove beyond the shadow of a doubt the many benefits of special diets or nutritional supplements for cancer patients undergoing chemotherapy and other mainstream treatments. You just have to know which ones are good and which ones are bad.

There is a great bias in mainstream medicine against using the diet to do anything other than alleviate the harmful side effects caused by mainstream therapies, and yet there are certain foods you should definitely avoid in your diet because they feed cancer or weaken your immune system, and others you should eat to help tackle cancer. Again, this is common sense. If you think of your diet as a cure, you can use your diet as a cancer remedy. But of course, you should not depend upon this alone.

Nevertheless, certain foods (or supplements) are *exactly* what you need to help fight cancer, since they attack it directly or strengthen your immune system so that it can do more fighting. Some types of nutrition will make you stronger or help to detoxify your body, which are especially important goals when you are undergoing various mainstream protocols such as chemotherapy. Better nutrition on your part will at the very least help to prevent cachexia (wasting syndrome), rebuild faulty cells and reduce the side effects of mainstream therapies, making them much easier for your body to handle. Better nutrition can help to buy you time for other treatments to work when your cancer is very aggressive. Your oncologist, whether mainstream or integrative, should want all these good things to happen.

As to nutritional supplements, while many doctors will tell you they are contraindicated for mainstream therapies, the truth for cancer patients is that you can definitely supplement most cancer treatments with specific vitamins, minerals and nutrient-rich foods or special supplements to get better outcomes. The *right* foods and nutraceutical supplements will not interfere with cancer treatments but can improve therapeutic results dramatically. The question is: which ones?

There are definitely special foods and nutritional items you can add to your diet to minimize the side effects of cancer treatments and maximize the process of getting well. Full spectrum vitamin E is an example of a simple supplement that protects against hair loss and heart damage when you undergo chemotherapy, and there are many more we could list (See Patrick Quillin's *Beating Cancer with Nutrition*). There are certain adjunctive foods and supplementary protocols that have even led to cancer cures on their own, although doctors dismissively call this a "spontaneous remission" when the recovery (even if it occurs on multiple patients) usually happens without the use of their conventional treatments.

To find out which ones are right for you, you should discuss the matter with cancer experts who commonly use these additional helpmates with their patients. This book just focuses on the main therapies and supplements typically producing the biggest impact for your efforts, but there are many others. We are only going to discuss the ones that will help you safely get started but typically produce *very noticeable* beneficial results. It would be sad indeed, with all this information available, if you ignored these therapies and started pinning your hopes on some obscure and unproven foods, supplements or protocols, when options with well-established efficacy are available.

This book emphasizes the 80/20 rule, which means that it focuses on just a few actionable things that are likely to have the greatest impact on your health. It does not bombard you with huge amounts of extraneous information that would not lead to major action steps or benefits. The world has certainly changed in that you can immediately look up any extra information you seek on the internet.

You need actionable steps that you can immediately take to help you get well, rather than yet another thick cancer book of "enlightening insights" and "interesting information" that doesn't motivate you to do anything. It therefore has exactly what you need to immediately get started with the extra powerful things you can do at home on your own without much worry or supervision.

SUPPLEMENTAL
CANCER
THERAPIES

3
THE BELJANSKI FORMULAS

The Beljanski herbal cancer formulas were invented by French-Serbian molecular biologist Mirko Beljanski Ph.D., whose story can be found in various books such as *Cancer's Cause, Cancer's Cure* by Dr. Morton Walker.

Dr. Walker wrote the following in the introduction to his book on the Beljanski botanical cancer formulas: "I have published ninety-one other books on consumer health, and I believe this book you're reading, number ninety-two, is my most momentous. I came out of retirement because I know that what Dr. Mirko Beljanski discovered could save millions of lives. His discoveries could put an end to the war on cancer."

In short, the importance of the Beljanski formulas is not something trivial. These formulas are at the top of the list of supplemental aids to be considered for many cancer patients.

During his 45 years of research, most of which were at the Pasteur Institute in France, Mirko Beljanski meticulously worked to isolate beneficial plant extracts for the treatment of cancer. These extracts, which work by selectively inhibiting the out-of-control replication of cancerous DNA while leaving normal cell DNA replication alone, have successfully reversed all kinds of cancer in Europe for patients at death's door or have prolonged survival for thousands of cancer patients.

In a tale filled with political intrigue and corruption, the French government seemed to disagree with this for various reasons, and threw him in jail at age 73 while confiscating all his notes and records. This occurred despite the effectiveness of his formulas, including the fact that they were even used by French President Francis Mitterrand.

The specific plant molecules Beljanksi discovered were alkaloid extracts from the African plant *Rauwolfia vomitoria* and a Brazilian rainforest tree, *Pao Pereira*. The two alkaloids have been definitively proven to inhibit the growth of cancer cells while leaving healthy cells alone. They kill cancer cells and only cancer cells, and they don't produce any inappropriate side effects at therapeutic levels. *Rauwolfia vomitoria* has a special affinity for endocrine/hormonal tissues while *Pao perira* attacks all cancer cells, can cross the blood brain barrier and is also a virus inhibitor.

This viral inhibition is important because of our previous discussion about HPV and other possible cancer microbes. There is even a microbial theory of cancer which proposes that microbes get inside healthy cells and thereby cause cancer; when they get inside the cell nucleus their DNA then mixes with the DNA of the cell, which then changes it. According to this theory, killing these microbes sometimes changes the unhealthy cells back to normal, thus stopping cancer in its tracks.

Many large cancer organizations will say that DNA damage causes cancer. Beljanski had found that many carcinogens did not mutate cellular DNA but simply interfered with the process of DNA replication. Therefore his botanical products set out to *fix the DNA replication process* when it ran amok, as happens with cancer. His botanicals supply limiting "bolt" molecules to the DNA transcription process, which has gone haywire in cancer cells, so these two extracts help stop cancer cells from replicating, while helping to restore DNA to a healthy state.

This approach is entirely different from *anything* offered by modern oncology and complements approaches such as chemo, surgery and radiation by trying to address the underlying problem. My naturopathic principle is to always attack a health problem using the redundancy of different synergistic approaches, which attack the problem from different angles. One of those unique directions is exactly what we have here, using an entirely non-toxic therapy with proven results.

Working at the level of repairing DNA replication mechanisms, their usage has resulted in many seemingly miraculous cancer cures. While they have often been known to produce cancer cures just on their own, studies have shown that when these botanical extracts are simultaneously coupled with traditional radiation and chemotherapy treatments, they *dramatically improve the effectiveness of these mainstream cancer therapies.* They reduce the side effects from these treatments and improve their therapeutic results. In some cases cure rates as high as 100% were achieved in animal studies that combined the Beljanski formulas with typical cancer treatments.

Today you can readily buy a combination of these two extracts in a Beljanski formula called "Prostabel." Prostabel serves as a basic self-help cancer supplement and can be used in conjunction with traditional cancer therapies. In addition to being a way to handle current cases of cancer, it is also used as an ongoing preventative, especially for individuals at high risk. Using Prostabel is as simple as swallowing a few pills at home. That's how easy it is to incorporate this into any anti-cancer regime.

Beljanksi formulated two other proven products for cancer patients that also enhance the effectiveness of traditional treatments. They are designed to reduce the normal side effects of conventional chemotherapy, surgery and radiation treatments, and thus are meant to work with these therapies. The first product, called "RealBuild," is made from the RNA fragments of non-pathogenic bacteria. These RNA primers activate bone marrow stem cells to produce more platelets and white blood cells in the body. The second product, called "Gingko V" extract, is produced from the golden leaf of the resilient and very ancient *Ginkgo biloba* tree. It protects against the typical harm caused by radiation therapy.

Beljanski developed his RNA fragments product, RealBuild, after noting that cancer chemotherapy and radiation treatment often caused a patent's level of blood platelets to drop so low that they sometimes bled to death during the course of treatment. While you can usually nutritionally reverse this condition by taking shark alkylglycerols (a simple fact most oncologists don't know), Beljanski also found that special RNA fragments led to the quick reappearance of new platelets in the blood and reversed low white blood cell counts by replacing those destroyed by chemotherapy. Therefore he developed these into a product for cancer patients.

Nutritionally speaking, to help preserve the bone marrow and its ability to make red and white blood cells, you might consider *eating bone marrow soup* and special botanicals to support their production. However, a much more reliable strategy is to use RNA fragments to help preserve the process of normal bone marrow cell replication. The result will definitely be a quicker proven increase in platelet and white cell production for cancer patients. This is a product you can definitely take on your own, and will have your doctor scratching his head wondering why your blood work is remaining so good when you are on chemo.

RNA fragments are to be taken when white blood cell and platelet levels fall to reduced levels due to radiation or chemotherapy, and are typically taken the day before any treatments begin. The RNA fragments are powders taken sublingually 2-3 times per week, and you avoid drinking liquids immediately after ingestion.

Black cumin oil (*Nigella sativa*), which is a Middle Eastern immunostimulant used for thousands of years, has also been discovered to increase bone marrow cells by 250%. Additionally, it has strong anti-bacterial and anti-inflammatory properties. It is an extremely inexpensive adjunct to any type of cancer protocol, including chemotherapy, since it also destroys cancer cells and inhibits tumor growth by as much as 50%.

In terms of helping cancer patients undergoing radiation therapy, Beljanski also worked to find a formula that might help cancer patients bear its typical side effects. He noted that *Ginkgo biloba* trees were famously resistant to the radiation damage at the atomic bombing sites of Hiroshima and Nagasaki. He therefore researched the tree's radiation-protective abilities and then created an extract of the golden (not the more commonly available green) leaves of the Ginkgo tree for those undergoing radiation therapy.

This special Gingko extract ("Gingko V") helps patients undergoing conventional radiation therapy to *avoid radiation burns and severe fibrosis* during radiation treatment. It doesn't have any detrimental side effects and greatly protects and relieves patients from the fibrosis typically induced over time by radiation therapy. If you are already undergoing radiation therapy or you are due to receive it, then you should immediately consider this product. Supplementation of 400 IU/day of vitamin E during radiation therapy (A.C. Grace brand "Unique E") will also reduce the severity of radiation induced side effects.

All of Beljanski's products improve clinical outcomes and enable you to continue to use harsh therapies without stopping. They are not damaging, deadly or costly and do not deteriorate anyone's quality of life. They only improve matters, so what is there to object to?

Each bottle of product naturally has suggested dosages and usage instructions. However, for more information on the Beljanski formulas, such as how to use his products in more complicated protocols, you might care to reference:

> *The Secret to Long Life in Your DNA: The Beljanski Approach to Cellular Health*, Herve Janecek and Monique Beljanski.

> *Cancer's Cause, Cancer's Cure*, Morton Walker.

> *The Beljanski Anti-Cancer Remedies: Inside the Double Helix of DNA*, Morton Walker and Randall Walker.

4
CARNIVORA

A Venus flytrap extract for cancer patients, called "Carnivora," was first developed in the 1970s by oncological investigator Dr. Helmut Keller at Klinik Winnerhof of Bad Wiessee, Germany. Keller reasoned that the Venus flytrap (*Dionaea muscipula*), which is a carnivorous plant that eats insects, must have an advanced immune system because it is able to distinguish between its own cells and the insects it must digest.

He therefore began testing Venus flytrap extracts to determine whether they could digest various cancer cell proteins. Out of his investigations, he eventually patented a Venus flytrap extract named "Carnivora," which contains an active ingredient called plumbagin. Dr. Keller treated over 2,000 patients with Carnivora, and other doctors have extensively used it for cancer and countless other immune problems since then.

The active ingredient of Carnivora, plumbagin, has been found to be a powerful immune-stimulant that can stop abnormal cell growth and the proliferation of cancer cells. Overall, the many ingredients within the extract give it immune modulating abilities by *blocking certain malignant tumor protein-kinases*. It also contains anti-mitotic amino acids, promotes phagocytosis and provides broad-spectrum anti-microbial action. It is a broad immune-stimulant and accomplishes an entire set of anti-cancer activities that are not usually addressed through mainstream cancer treatments.

Carnivora is not used for cancer alone but for many types of immune compromised conditions. The extract has been found to be very beneficial for chronic infections and various types of degenerative disease. In particular, it has been used by *many celebrities* to treat their cancer, including Ronald Reagan, who used it after his surgery for colon cancer.

While Dr. Keller's cancer patient work has not appeared in peer-reviewed journals, this doesn't mean that Carnivora isn't effective. In 1985 Keller published a study in a German medical journal which claimed that out of 210 cancer cases, 56% of the patients experienced either remission or stabilization of their tumors after taking Carnivora. Whereas the results of this study have never been verified nevertheless, since that time Carnivora has been used quite successfully by many cancer doctors. They have consistently mentioned its effectiveness at helping produce tumor regression and in stabilizing cancer so that it does not worsen.

In addition to Keller's research, the Chief of Oncopharmacology at the National Oncological Center of Bulgaria, Professor D.K. Todorov, M.D., Ph.D., D.Sc., performed clinical studies on Carnivora for over two decades, conducting cancer research at Heidelberg University in Germany. His *in vitro* research found that cancer cells from various cell lines were destroyed within hours when exposed to Carnivora! Because of these *in vitro* findings, some doctors started using the extract *in vivo*, treating patients with sarcoma tumors. Despite previous treatment with toxic therapies, some patients achieved complete remission after relying on just this product alone.

The Institute of Pharmaceutical Biology of the University of Munich also found that Carnivora *decreases the ATP content of cells*. In depressing the energy of malignant cells, this causes them to weaken over a relatively short period of time, which in turn makes them more susceptible to elimination by the body's immune system. Two other popular cancer-fighting botanicals, Graviola and Paw Paw, work in a similar way by lowering the ATP energy within cancer cells so that they eventually fall apart. Paw Paw has even been shown effective against multiple drug resistant (MDR) cancer cells while many MDR lines are also sensitive to curcumin, but it is not yet known whether Carnivora, which works on similar principles to Paw Paw, shares this same characteristic.

Most alternative cancer therapies work because of unique scientific principles like this that approach cancer from entirely different angles than what is used in mainstream oncology. The pharmaceutical perspective doesn't like to admit that natural botanicals can have such effects, and yet botanicals have been used to successfully treat diseases like cancer for thousands of years. Carnivora basically works against cancer by stripping the outer protein shell of cancer cells and then gradually depleting the ATP inside of these abnormal cells.

This unique *modus operandi*, which isn't shared by mainstream cancer strategies, is just another example that indicates why you should consider using multiple supplemental therapies to treat any medical condition, because you don't know which angle of approach will work best. *The ability to simultaneously attack a disease on different fronts from different angles, using entirely different methods,* will usually give you better chances of recovery than if you rely on just a single line of approach alone that may not work, and the earlier you get started at this the better. That is why this book on supplemental, synergistic cancer therapies was written, for the goal is to help you attack cancer from as many different directions possible at the same time so that you maximize the possible outcome from any mainstream or other treatment regimen you decide upon.

Studies performed at the KTB Tumor Research Institute at the Institute of Molecular Medicine and Tumor Biology, Germany, also found that Carnivora would selectively attack cancer cells by inhibiting their mitochondrial ATP synthesis and by interfering with protein kinase production, thus resulting in apoptosis (programmed cell death). Basically, certain enzymes within Carnivora block various proteins in tumorous cancer cells. When blocked, the cancer cells subsequently die off, which results in cell apoptosis. Carnivora also supports macrophage production and activity by stimulating phagocytosis, which comes in to help clean up all the cellular lysing debris that is produced when cancer cells destruct.

Researchers at Zytognost GmbH in Munich, Germany, reported that Venus Flytrap juice decreased suppressor cells while increasing helper cells. This result modulates the body's entire immune system by increasing the efficiency of the helper/suppressor cell (CD4/CD8) ratio, thereby producing a more effective immune response. Persons treated with Carnivora also show significant increases in natural killer cells, as demonstrated in clinical studies performed since the 1970's. In studying its use to combat HIV, research found that Carnivora extract would attack pathogenic organisms, kill them, digest their toxins, and leave behind dead microbial remains for removal from the patient's bloodstream by phagocytosis.

All these various results are exactly what we want!

In summary, you cannot say that Carnivora has not been studied or that it does not work in fighting cancer. Countless health practitioners have proven otherwise, and especially doctors in Germany, who are certainly no fools. Carnivora has been used for over thirty years, especially within Europe, for its multi-faceted ability to modulate/enhance the entire immune system and for its specific ability to fight cancer. It is an immune modulator used to help prevent cancer or actively battle against cancer. It is typically used as a supplemental nutrient because it is helpful in most immune deficiency conditions, showing anti-microbial activity against many bacteria, viruses and other internal pathogens. Therefore if you want to help prevent opportunistic infections when you have cancer, just for this one reason alone the product should be considered.

In short, Carnivora has been used by itself or in conjunction with other therapies for the treatment of both cancer and non-cancerous diseases. It is safe; it has no toxic side effects and does not harm healthy, normal cells. You can even use it on pets. There are no known contraindications with any prescription drugs or other dietary supplements. However, while there are no known contraindications for any other drugs or therapies, as with all supplements you should check with your physician before using Carnivora, especially if you are pregnant or on blood thinner medications.

Over time, Carnivora extract has become more and more used as a popular supplemental cancer treatment. Do not expect it to cure you, but you can expect to feel better after using it since this is what people commonly report. While in some cases there have been complete cancer remissions for some users, it is just considered another supplemental helpmate for cancer that works along a different set of healing principles than those utilized by chemotherapy, surgery and radiation.

To its credit, there are many testimonials reporting that Carnivora shrinks tumors and works well for most types of cancer, although it is most effective for cancers that are characterized as early and intermediate. It is also used for the maintenance of an efficient immune system in general, which is important during remission. The basic method for fighting an immune disease is to take dried herb capsules or a liquid extract several times throughout the day.

Like most supplemental aids, Carnivora is the most effective when other dietary and lifestyle factors are also addressed at the same time, and when it is part of a larger set of supplemental therapies that might include activities such as vegetable juicing, lymph drainage and various DMSO/MSM protocols. It is often used together with other immune-stimulating herbs such as Cat's Claw or Pau d'arco and is said to work best when a cancer patient has not previously undergone chemotherapy or radiation therapy.

You can find out more about Carnivora in Dr. Morton Walker's *Natural Cancer Remedies That Work*. The product is available in liquid extract or capsule form, which represent different potencies, and can easily be used as a dietary supplement to maintain a healthy immune system. Carnivora.com is a well-known manufacturer whose product quality can be depended upon. The dosage to be used depends on a variety of factors, including the type of disease, the patient's condition and as stated, whether the individual has previously undergone other therapies, such as chemo or radiation.

Whether using either capsules or liquid extract, to avoid feeling a Herxheimer die-off reaction you must start using Carnivora slowly and only gradually work up to a higher dosage. Because Carnivora kills most types of pathogens within the body as well as cancer cells, a short-term die-off reaction can occur if you start taking too much too soon. A Herxheimer reaction simply proves that a substance is indeed destroying internal pathogens, which are the precursors of disease, and is due to the fact that the body cannot eliminate the toxins fast enough. It becomes so inundated with cellular debris that its detoxification systems get temporarily overloaded. Nobody experiences a Herxheimer reaction if they build up usage gradually.

Carnivora extract capsules, which are typically used by early or intermediate stage cancer patients, work to wake up the body's immune system in a multi-faceted way. While they work against all sorts of internal pathogens including cancer, you should not consider the capsules as being strong enough to battle cancer by themselves. They are a supplement used by people who simply want to help boost and then maintain their immune system so that they can stay healthy. While you are undergoing chemotherapy, your immune system typically becomes severely damaged while both cancer *and normal cells* are adversely affected. Carnivora works against *just cancer cells,* leaving normal cells alone, while helping your immune system to maintain its strength. Liquid Carnivora extract is stronger than the dried extract and is especially used for advanced immune conditions, such as late stage cancer.

You should not take Carnivora capsules and extracts at the same time but should alternate between them. Most people don't know that most herbal liquid extracts lose their efficacy if taken on a daily basis, and Carnivora follows this principle as well. You can avoid the loss of potency (effectiveness) that occurs with all extracts by alternating the use of capsule and liquid concentrate. For instance, you can take the stronger liquid extract daily Monday through Saturday (or any other set of six consecutive days per week) and then switch to using capsules on Sunday. Every fifth week you should not use the liquid extract at all, but simply take the capsules instead. In other words, abstaining from Carnivora extract every five weeks will help to preserve its efficacy, so every fifth week you should replace Carnivora liquid extract by using dried extract capsules instead.

Information on Carnivora is readily found within many cancer publications. The only thing that publications usually don't mention is that it can be safely used for a cat or dog who gets cancer, which is yet another reason to look into it and consider it as a supplemental aid.

Natural Cancer Remedies That Work, Morton Walker.

Cancer: Step Outside the Box, Ty Bollinger.

German Cancer Therapies: Natural and Conventional Medicines that Offer Hope and Healing, Morton Walker.

Alternative Medicine Definitive Guide to Cancer, W. John Diamond and W. Lee Cowden.

5

SPECIAL COLLOIDAL MINERALS

Many platinum-based chemotherapy agents, such as cisplatin and carboplatin, rely on the properties of platinum for fighting cancer. The molecular basis of their effectiveness is that platinum can chemically bond with DNA and can, through this mechanism, inhibit the growth and replication of cancer cells in the body. Cisplatin and carboplatin, which are the components of many chemotherapy protocols, were originally manufactured by Johnson Matthey scientists and are particularly used for the treatment of ovarian and testicular cancers.

Here is why platinum is the basis of many chemotherapy drugs. When platinum is present in a cell, only one of the DNA helices is affected. By a mechanism that is not well understood at this time, the platinum locates and binds to the damaged helix. The platinum that is present within the cell then interferes with the mitotic cycle of cell division (mitosis). Platinum binds to the cell's DNA in a very specific way that creates a tiny kink in the DNA strand, and this imperfection stops the rapid cell division of tumor growth. This is how it combats cancer.

While other metals can also produce a kink in the DNA, only the presence of platinum produces the perfect timing balance during mitosis that halts the division and thus proliferation of tumor cells. Basically, platinum disrupts the mitosis cycle of cell replication so that a cancerous cell does not continue to divide out of control. Eventually, the platinum atom naturally leaves the DNA strand and is then excreted from the body.

Is there a less toxic way of delivering platinum to the body other than through the path of toxic chemotherapy?

Yes, there is the possibility of drinking *colloidal platinum* on an empty stomach, whereby the platinum nanoparticles will be directly absorbed into the bloodstream via the digestive tract and then eventually picked up by the cancer cells. This delivers platinum molecules to your body via the digestive tract (you just drink it), rather than intravenously.

Unfortunately, no pharmaceutical company wants to research the cancer fighting properties of pure colloidal platinum because there is no money to be made. Since platinum is an element it cannot be patented, so the pharmaceutical industry cannot generate any great monopolistic revenues from this approach. In order to get a patent, pharmaceutical firms must complex simple platinum with an organic molecule that is far larger than a platinum nanoparticle and thus harder to get into a cancer cell.

Even though colloidal platinum is not a patented pharmaceutical, many cancer patients have seen their cancer disappear by drinking this liquid, and appreciate the fact that colloidal platinum is similar to chemotherapy in respect of its way of working. This is not the same as chemotherapy and it is not a replacement for chemotherapy. However, it doesn't destroy your immune system and unlike chemotherapy, it causes no uncomfortable side effects in delivering platinum to cancer cells.

Only one company produces a true colloidal platinum product of nanometer-sized particles, which is the most absorbable form of any metal or mineral supplement, and that company is Purest Colloids of Westampton, New Jersey (PurestColloids.com). Its platinum nanoparticles are only 37 times larger than the diameter of a single platinum atom, which is the smallest in the industry. The smaller the size of the particle, the easier it can be absorbed into cells and so become an active agent.

Purest Colloids produces various colloidal minerals through a special process that maximizes the colloidal nature of the product while minimizing the ionic content of the beverages. This special process is beyond the technological capabilities of most other colloidal mineral manufacturers, which is why the company can produce the smallest sized colloidal mineral particles in the world. Because of such small nanoparticles, the Purest

Colloids products maximize the important surface area to mass ratio of the particles within them.

As with all colloidal mineral manufacturers, Purest Colloids does not sell or advertise any of its products as a treatment for cancer, nor does it market any of its products as effective against cancer or any other disease. It simply sells colloidal minerals that people use for health reasons. Various colloidal mineral products have been used by people for years throughout the world, and are often used by cancer patients as a complement to other therapies.

Colloidal silver is of special interest along these lines because it is employed in many anti-microbial therapies for numerous immune conditions, cancer being just one of them. Some of the most popular colloidal silver brands include Utopia Silver, ASAP Plus, as well as the MesoSilver brand produced by Purest Colloids, whose silver nanoparticles are just 2.6 times the diameter of a single silver atom.

Colloidal silver attacks all viruses, bacteria, fungi, mycoplasmas, amoeba and other microbial pathogens within the body. This is a very important result for those who have been on high sugar diets, which in particular feeds yeast (fungi) in the body. As previously mentioned, Candisol/Candex is one particular supplement used to help with yeast infections. As for colloidal silver, it is not an immune stimulant but an anti-microbial agent that lowers the overall pathogenic burden on the immune system. In attacking many different types of microbial invaders, it consequently boosts your immune strength because it lowers your internal pathogenic load.

By killing microbes, colloidal silver frees up your immune system so it can devote its energies to combatting cancer, rather than remain preoccupied with primarily attacking pathogens. It does not fight cancer directly but helps by reducing infectious agents, which is especially helpful when your immune system has been severely compromised by cancer or traditional therapies such as chemo. Colloidal silver has basically been used by hundreds of thousands of people for decades to help eliminate various infections that are burdening their immune system.

You absolutely want this result when you are fighting cancer. As an adjunctive supplement, colloidal silver therefore helps cancer patients fight off opportunistic infections when they are undergoing various cancer treatments such as radiation, chemotherapy or other therapies. Some nutritional supplements stimulate the immune system so that it becomes supercharged to better fight cancer and internal microbes, whereas colloidal silver just goes right in and kills pathogenic invaders directly.

As previously mentioned, some researchers believe that certain types of cancer are even caused by viral or bacterial pathogens ("cancer microbes"), and if this is true then it is yet another reason why you would want various supplemental strategies, such as colloidal silver nanoparticles, to attack these microbes directly.

Various nutrient protocols aimed at treating cancer, such as the Budwig diet protocol or Gerson therapy, do not address cancer from the microbial angle because they work via an entirely different *modus operandi*. That is why I like to stack various supplemental therapies together for any health condition. With colloidal silver, we must consider the following: if a substance kills any pathogens that play a role in the "pathogenic theory of cancer," we would then have to say that it is attacking one potential root cause of the problem.

On the internet, various cancer protocols can easily be found that use colloidal silver together with concentrated forms of organic sulfur (in the form of MSM or DMSO) to help silver nanoparticles kill any microbes in the bloodstream, penetrate cell membranes to kill any pathogens that may be inside cells, and thereby build up the immune system. However, the extra MSM/DMSO is not necessary when using MesoSilver because of the already extremely small particle size of this brand of colloidal silver. If you visualize a silver nanoparticle as being the size of a BB then a cell wall membrane would look like a basketball net, and at that scale the cell wall membranes are very porous and therefore virtually irrelevant. Thus when using this brand there is no reason for organic sulfur to help make cell membranes more permeable for silver's absorption.

CancerTutor.com publishes quite a few colloidal silver/DMSO protocols on its website that may be helpful when you use other brands of colloidal silver with larger nanoparticles. It may also be true that the sulfur in these protocols is helpful for reasons other than increasing cellular permeability, as Dr. Budwig discovered when she created her own flax oil/cottage cheese protocol that relies on sulfurated proteins. In this case the sulfur-containing proteins help make dietary lipids more water-soluble so that they can travel throughout the body and reach the cells requiring them for repair.

Cesium is another metal used in alternative cancer treatments, via cesium chloride protocols, to attack tumors by accumulating inside their cells. When the highly alkaline cesium enters cancer cells it changes their metabolism. It makes them dysfunctional so that they can no longer feed or reproduce themselves. Yet another non-mainstream product (Poly-MVA) uses the metals/minerals palladium, molybdenum, rhodium and ruthenium along with alpha-lipoic acid in a special mixture to target cancer cell gene repair mechanisms while leaving normal, healthy cells alone. Calcium is used in other naturopathic protocols to help alkalize the body against cancer, too.

All these examples prove that pure minerals and metals can be and are used in various cancer treatments. However, no one knows for certain whether it is a metal/mineral's ability to enter a cancer cell or its ability to kill microbes that is helping most; it is hard to differentiate which ability is attacking a cause of cancer or a result of cancer. For instance, some researchers speculate that the DNA of microbes within cancer cells might be the very thing that damages the DNA of a normal cell and causes cancer. Along this line of thinking, when a metal/mineral enters a cancer cell and causes destruction, does it help eliminate cancer because it is killing harmful cancer-causing microbes within the cell or is the metal/mineral producing biochemical changes that cause a cell to self-destruct or revert back to normal? All anyone currently knows for sure is that there are ways of using various metals and minerals (platinum, silver, cesium, gold, etc.) that often produce highly beneficial results against tumors because they act upon different mechanisms. The results are what counts.

The producer of the smallest sized colloidal mineral products on the market is definitely Purest Colloids which, like all other colloidal mineral manufacturers and all the distributors of the other products mentioned in this book, does not sell or advertise any of its product as a treatment for cancer, nor does it market any of its products as effective against cancer or any other disease. It simply sells colloidal minerals that people all over the world use for health reasons.

One particular combination product of interest, called "Meso-SGPS," combines colloidal platinum, silver and gold in effective proportions. It combines three cancer-fighting metals together. Platinum addresses DNA replication errors, silver addresses microbial infections in the body (or within cancer cells, as some have claimed) and colloidal gold addresses anti-angiogenesis. Colloidal gold has strong anti-angiogenesis properties, which means it can help to reduce the growth of new blood vessels around tumors.

The typical dosage of this combination product is one ounce of liquid taken four times per day. Because colloidal copper is also beneficial but cannot be combined in the same colloidal suspension, it is typically taken separately at the same time. The typical dosage is one tablespoon four times per day. In other words, individuals with immune problems usually take separate tablespoons of colloidal platinum, silver, gold and copper four times per day, or they take one ounce of Meso-SGPS along with one tablespoon of colloidal copper four times per day.

Is this a cure for cancer? Hardly. However, you can say that it addresses various cancer issues from different angles that may be contributory to your health, and the colloidal silver component definitely will lower internal burdens on your immune system. It will provide assistance when you most need it, which is a great boon when your immune system is already compromised by the burden of cancer or when it has been destroyed by chemotherapy.

Further information on the ability of platinum-based pharmaceutical compounds to treat cancer, on colloidal silver products for attacking infections, and on colloidal minerals in general can be readily found on the internet.

6

DR. JOANNA BUDWIG'S FLAXSEED OIL AND COTTAGE CHEESE MIXTURE

We are revisiting the Budwig flaxseed oil and cottage cheese (FOCC) combination because many oncologists consider this food item a key dietary component in any cancer treatment. They may propose entirely different diets to help you get well, but they will typically ask patients to include the famous Budwig flaxseed oil and cottage cheese mixture in whatever diet they use. It is both a preventative and curative food item. You will also shortly see that the majority of the other Budwig diet principles, such as avoiding sugar, are commonly shared by most anti-cancer diets, too.

The famous Budwig flaxseed oil and cottage cheese mixture is not just a dietary item, but a cancer protocol in itself because it has a known history of eliminating cancer. Literally thousands of people have claimed that they owe their life to this very simple food. In 1990 the oncologist Dr. Dan C. Roehm re-examined Budwig's basic diet using the FOCC formula and declared, "This diet is far and away the most successful anti-cancer diet in the world."

Even so, the Budwig FOCC mixture and diet takes time to work, so it is not a quick curative aid. Cancer patients might need 3-6 months before they see tumors shrink although other health conditions they might have may respond much faster. Budwig pointed out that cancer patients who start on the protocol and get their cancer under control must also continue with a maintenance dose (of one tablespoon of flaxseed oil per one hundred pounds of body weight) to prevent remission, but this assumes that they did not use any other therapies than her diet to get well.

The famous FOCC combination can certainly be added to your diet whether you are undergoing surgery, radiation or chemotherapy. It cannot hurt but can only help. In fact, Budwig warned that the mainstream protocols by themselves would likely hurt you, especially chemotherapy. In any case, you are going to be using organic flaxseed oil combined with organic cottage cheese to build better cell membranes that will, as a result, help cure cancer. The formula can be used for other chronic diseases, too.

So who was Dr. Joanna Budwig and why does the flaxseed oil and cottage cheese mixture work? What exactly does it do?

Dr. Budwig was Germany's Senior Expert for fats and pharmaceutical drugs in the Central Government and was considered one of the world's leading authorities on fats and oils. Her research basically proved that commercially processed fats and oils (hydrogenated or partially hydrogenated fats) weaken or destroy cellular membranes and consequently lower the electrical potential within body cells, which often then leads to chronic or terminal illness.

When we digest fats, our bodies break them down into their component building block pieces called "fatty acids." Fatty acids are important to our physiology because when you remove the water from our bodies, more than 50% of what's left is fatty acids. If we consume "bad fats" that are deficient in some way because of commercial processing, we cannot build strong cells that function properly because the fatty acids used to build new cells will be deficient. In essence, eating too many commercially processed fats supplies poor building materials for our cells because the processing destroys the vital electron clouds of those fats. Eating these damaged fats over time, which are then incorporated into the many cells of the body, eventually causes a shut down of the electrical field of those cells. After a sufficient tipping point, chronic or terminal disease can then eventually set in. However, this can be reversed if we start supplying our bodies with the right type of fats.

Our cells have a negatively charged outer membrane and a positively charged inner nucleus. The electrically negative cell membrane is composed to a large extent of unsaturated fatty acids. These fatty acids carry oxygen into our cells, so we can say that they are responsible for cellular respiration. Dr. Otto Warburg won a Nobel Prize in part for studying cellular respiration, and discovered that the anaerobic energy generation mechanism within cancer cells was a consequence of damaged or insufficient cellular respiration. His research therefore introduced the now popular idea that cancer cells thrive in anaerobic environments without oxygen.

Continuing along this line of thought, Budwig found that when the electrons have been removed from the fatty acids of our cells, they can no longer bind with oxygen which, in turn, then inhibits cellular respiration and favors the development of cancer. Healthy omega-3 fats in the diet, however, help defeat cancer by supplying the right fatty acids that rejuvenate cellular membranes so that their oxygenation mechanism is restored and the cancer cells can start breathing again! Studies of a famous anti-cancer product called "Ukrain" show that when you increase the oxygen consumption of cancer cells it tends to overwhelm them, effectively killing them. Basically, high oxygen tension tends to be lethal to cancer cells. Since you definitely start increasing the cellular oxygenation of cancer cells when you use the FOCC mixture to restore good fatty acids to the body that then slowly replace the depleted fatty acids used to build those faulty cells, this helps to explain why Budwig's formula has led to so many cancer "cures" or "remissions." It should be part of every cancer patient's diet.

The right fatty acids will start effecting repairs everywhere within the body, which is why they start to reverse all sorts of degenerative conditions. However, Dr. Emanuel Revici, who designed highly effective cancer treatments for patients using lipids or lipid-like synthetic compounds, found that lipids have an affinity for cancer tumors and thus are readily taken up by them. This may help explain why the Budwig fatty acid protocol is so effective at targeting cancer, although it also works at correcting many other health problems, too. Revici also differed from Budwig in that he only used fatty acid supplementation when he found cancer patients were producing an excess of sterols in their bodies, and gave sterols and other agents to cancer patients when their bodies were producing a predominance of fatty acids. This is a key hint for more research in this area.

Unfortunately, in our diets we have slowly been replacing pure unsaturated fats with chemically treated unsaturated fats, and thus supplying our bodies with *damaged fatty acids* that are electron cloud deficient. They are unable to easily perform all the activities of cellular respiration. When an unsaturated fat undergoes chemical processing, its surrounding field of electrons is altered. If those amputated fats then become the primary source of fats that the body receives, our bodies will start using the crippled fatty acids to build new cells because they are the only thing available. However, the cell membranes of those new cells will be very weak because of this underlying deficiency. These weak cell membranes, with damaged electron fields, then become *the first biochemical step toward cancer*.

The field of electrons surrounding fatty acids is important for the optimal functioning of all sorts of biochemical processes wherever the fats are used within the human body. Cell membranes in our bodies need this outer field of electrons to grow and function properly, but as stated their energy fields will be damaged if your diet lacks the right sorts of fats. If you continually consume dietary fats that have been deadened because their electrons have been removed, the bioelectrical action for all sorts of cellular functions in your body will gradually be affected, especially cellular respiration. Various functions will get "locked up" and slow down or stop working, which can lead to disease.

As the wrong types of fatty acids in cell membranes become predominant everywhere, more and more cells will slow down or become paralyzed and your entire body will show a loss of electrical potential. Next, some sort of chronic disease or fatal condition such as cancer is likely to set in. Only if you add the right lipids (fats) to the diet can this degradation be reversed and your health restored.

This process even ties into the events of cellular mitosis. During the process of cellular division to grow new cells, the mother and daughter cells must both contain enough electron-rich fatty acids in the cell's surface area so that there can be a complete division of the new daughter cell from the mother cell, and one cell can become two. If the electron-rich fatty acids are not present in the cell's surface area, the dipolarity between the cell membrane and cell nucleus will decrease and possibly disappear. The complex will then become inactive and cells will begin to die before the maturing and splitting process of the cells ever takes place. Budwig stated that this is the reason that tumors form.

How do you reverse this? Dr. Budwig found that if you provide the body with a very simple food, which is the famous cottage cheese and flax seed oil (FOCC) combination, this can supply the right electron-rich fatty acids that will rejuvenate the stagnated growth processes and slowly restore things to normal. Supplying your body with the right type of fats/lipids, which contain the right types of cellular building materials, will also *naturally cause tumors within the body to dissolve* as depleted fatty acids are replaced with electron-rich good fatty acids. Consequently, a whole range of biochemical "dead battery" symptoms (due to the depleted electron fields) will then be cured.

The question then is, "Why these two particular ingredients?"

Budwig found that flaxseed oil was extremely rich in the essential electron-rich unsaturated fats we need for health. Cottage cheese, on the other hand, is rich in sulfur-containing ("sulfurated") proteins. The chemical reaction between the two, when mixed, *makes the fats water-soluble*. This allows them to become more free-flowing throughout the body and more easily absorbed into cells.

It's just a fact of physical chemistry that fats are only water-soluble and free-flowing in the body when they are bound to protein, so Budwig essentially found a simple way to mix two foods together so that the essential fatty acids could be much more readily absorbed into the body. In particular, Budwig wanted sulfurated proteins (containing methionine and cysteine) and a highly unsaturated but electron-rich fat that could be a large electron donor. When electron-rich fats are combined with proteins, the valuable electrons are protected until the body requires energy, upon which this energy source is tapped on demand.

If you can find another highly unsaturated but electron-rich fatty acid source other than flaxseed oil, this would also work. If you could find another way to make the fats more water soluble other than using sulfurated proteins, or find an alternative source of sulfurated proteins other than cottage cheese, this would work, too. For instance, foods containing protein compounds with a high sulfur content include cheese, nuts, egg yolks, asparagus, onions and the Alium family of vegetables (leeks, chives and garlic), *but most especially cottage cheese*. Some of these foods contain only low levels of sulfurated proteins, which is what we need to make the oil water-soluble.

Incidentally, supplements with a high sulfur content include alpha lipoic acid, chlorella, DMSO/MSM, NAC, cysteine, glutathione and even turmeric, which should be added to the diet for other reasons. It is amazing how often we see the same foods and supplements appearing again and again on different lists of items that are useful for fighting cancer.

The electron-rich unsaturated fats you should be seeking in your diet are usually the linoleic fats, which include flaxseed, sunflower, safflower, soybean, poppyseed, evening primrose and walnut oils as well as others. Their molecular structure supports a rich field of electrons that stores an electrical charge that can be conducted off into the body as necessary, thus recharging cells and tissues. Basically, the molecular and electron structure of these fats *help improve all the cells of the body*, which plays a role in beating cancer.

It would actually be a highly admirable research project for a physical chemist to design an alternative to the FOCC mixture that would help cancer patients along these same lines. However, so far no one has taken on the task. Dr. Emanuel Revici (see *The Doctor Who Cures Cancer* by William Eidem) won renown in curing thousands of cancer patients because he used his physical chemistry background to develop a way of encasing high doses of selenium with a lipid coating so that it could be safely absorbed into cancer cells and dissolve them from within. It seems that physical chemists have the skills to develop particularly powerful anti-cancer therapies.

Let's get down to the step-by-step process for actually producing the FOCC mixture at home. To prepare the cottage cheese and flaxseed oil combo to eat, you will need two appliances: an immersion stick hand-held blender and a coffee bean grinder to grind flaxseeds. Once you have everything ready, in a bowl you combine two or more tablespoons of organic cottage cheese with one tablespoon of flaxseed oil, and then blend the mixture at *slow speed* for about one minute using the immersion blender. This mixing ratio is key: *two tablespoons of cottage cheese to about one tablespoon of oil*. For example, you might mix four tablespoons of cottage cheese with two tablespoons of flaxseed oil. You can use organic full-fat goat's milk cottage cheese instead of low-fat cow's milk cottage cheese in order to avoid dairy.

You stop blending when the mixture develops a creamy texture, like whipped cream, with no separated oil. This usually requires about a minute or more of immersion blender mixing. Hand mixing will not blend the two substances sufficiently, so a key is the blending with an immersion blender, rather than by hand, so that the oil and cottage cheese can bond. The sulfurated proteins in the cottage cheese must make contact with the oil so that it becomes water soluble, allowing it to then be easily digested and assimilated into the cells of the body. You can find a great Youtube video by Sandra Olsen showing the simple mixing procedure: "Budwig Diet Flaxseed and Cottage Cheese."

How often should you eat the combo? It depends on the severity of your condition. Most people usually start slowly by eating FOCC just once a day, and then work their way up to eating more often so that their bodies can adjust. A typical schedule is to eat it at least twice per day. Budwig pointed out that people who were suffering from a terminal disease like cancer should work up to consuming 4-8 tablespoons of the oil daily.

You can also add other foods to the mixture to make it tastier, but only after it has already been mixed! For instance, you can sprinkle 1-2 tablespoons of freshly ground flax seed over the top of the freshly mixed FOCC mixture to supercharge it, or you can even mix it in by hand. Flaxseed goes rancid within 15-20 minutes after grinding, so eat the mixture right away. Furthermore, don't ever use pre-ground flaxseed but grind it fresh with a small coffee grinder right before eating. Store the seeds in your refrigerator and grind them fresh each time, mixing them in by hand immediately after the initial blending.

You can also stir in (not more than one cup of) nuts, banana, organic cocoa, cinnamon, vanilla, organic shredded coconut, fresh pineapple, blueberries and raspberries or other fresh organic fruit. A more common way of eating these extras is to place them on top of the completed mixture, rather than stirring them together. That's what I do, and adding extras makes it taste great.

Some people think that they are using the Budwig protocol if they substitute yogurt for the cottage cheese, but this does not work. Only cottage cheese (or quark) contains the sulfurated protein that is the basis of the Budwig formula and the reason why it works. The flaxseed oil should also be kept refrigerated so that it does not go rancid. Dr. Budwig stressed the need to follow her program in an exact manner, warning that otherwise the results would probably be disappointing.

As to the rest of the Budwig diet, as stated it follows many of the same dietary principles we have already gone over and commonly find in other diets: Here is what you avoid:

- White sugar, molasses or maple syrup – sugar is absolutely forbidden in the diet
- Ice cream or dairy products (except the cottage cheese or quark used in the protocol)
- Trans-fats and hydrogenated oils such as margarine, salad oils and mayonnaise (use cold-pressed linoleic oils instead such as extra virgin olive oil, sunflower seed oil, etc.)
- White flour products (bread, pasta, …) but whole grain is allowed
- Soy products (unless fermented); corn is discouraged
- Processed foods, pesticides and chemicals
- Microwave, teflon or aluminum cookware (use enamelware, CorningWare, stainless steel, ceramic or glass cooking ware instead)
- Pork and animal fats
- Bottom feeding seafood or filter-feeding seafood that is known to collect and concentrate toxins and heavy metals (lobsters, clams, shrimp, mussels, etc.)

Freshly squeezed juices (ex. carrot, red beets, apple, etc.) are fine on a Budwig diet, and three times per day a warm tea is also recommended. This can even be Essiac, Pau d'arco or other teas known to help fight cancer. However, Dr. Budwig often warned against using her protocol in conjunction with other therapies that could go against the benefits of her formula, and this includes laetrile, bio-oxidative therapies or vitamin C infusions.

Here's the short of it. By eating a combination of two simple foods that are blended together, sometimes cancer can be cured. If not, this omega-3 mixture will still certainly contribute to building healthier cells, improving internal biochemical processes and reducing inflammation. It will help the body restore cellular respiration to normal. Unrefined, cold-pressed flaxseed oil doesn't work well by itself, but is the best oil for the FOCC mixture.

As usual, the mainstream medical establishment commonly says that there is no research supporting the use of the FOCC mixture, readily ignoring thousands of documented testimonials and the science behind the formula. Nonetheless, it is one of the most important supplemental aids you can use in getting well. Budwig would even take extremely sick cancer patients from the hospital with only days to live, and using this protocol along with special oil enemas would often even cure them.

You can easily add this supplemental therapy to your diet. Information on the Budwig cottage cheese and flaxseed oil mixture is readily found on the internet and in such books as:

FlaxOil as a True Aid Against Arthritis, Heart Infarction, Cancer and Other Diseases, Dr. Joanna Budwig.

Cancer – The Problem and the Solution, Dr. Joanna Budwig.

The Oil-Protein Diet Cookbook, Dr. Joanna Budwig.

A Day in the Budwig Diet: The Book: Learn Dr. Budwig's Complete Home Healing Protocol Against Cancer, Arthritis, Heart Disease & More, Ursual Escher.

Cancer-Free: Your Guide to Gentle, Non-toxic Healing, Bill Henderson.

7
OJIBWA OR ESSIAC TEA

One of the simplest adjunctive therapy recommendations for cancer patients is that they start drinking green tea. Green tea is helpful because it contains special polyphenols that induce programmed cell death (apoptosis) in cancer cells.

As you know, cancer cells cannot handle oxygen but thrive on glucose metabolism instead. This is why a cancer patient should dramatically cut sugar from their diet since that sugar will actually feed the cancer calls. Even though this is the case, you will often find hospitals feeding you candy and cookies in the chemotherapy room!

Here is the extent of the problem. A hundred years ago the average person ate less than four pounds of sugar per year, but now we are eating more than 170 pounds per annum. This extremely high sugar level in the diet, especially within sugary drinks, is one of the reasons behind the large surges seen in obesity, diabetes and cancer rates across the world. Our high sugar consumption is feeding these sicknesses.

Feeding your cancer while simultaneously trying to kill it is suicidal behavior. Since any cancer patient who drinks sweet liquids, such as soda or milk, is feeding their cancer cells and promoting their growth, this is another reason you should switch to drinking green tea instead. Green tea polyphenols don't just induce cancer cell death but also inhibit tumor proliferation and tumor blood vessel growth factors. Cellular biologist Dr.

Stephen Hsu also found that these polyphenols destroyed the mitochondria of cancer cells, which provide them with energy.

The most abundant anti-cancer ingredient in green tea is epigallocatechin gallate, commonly referred to as EGCG. This substance binds to a protein found on tumor cells and inhibits their growth. Specifically, EGCG binds to and neutralizes BCL-XL, also known as the anti-death protein found in a cancer cell that does not allow the cell to die. Because of BCL-XL, cancer cells reproduce quickly and are resistant to being killed with chemotherapy and/or radiation treatments. EGCG, however, inserts itself into a crevice found on the surface of the BCL-XL molecule and blocks its activity, permitting cellular death.

Green tea supplements typically have high levels of EGCG, and these are the supplements most often used in the mainstream medical trials showing positive outcomes for cancer patients undergoing chemotherapy or radiation (or both). What research has discovered is that mainstream treatments *are usually much more effective and have fewer side effects when green tea high in EGCG is used together with them,* probably because it takes less poison to kill cells when EGCG is present. Thus, this is a perfect supplemental therapy!

If you have any type of cancer, the least you can do is to stop drinking sugary drinks and instead start drinking green tea with a high EGCG content. You might also take EGCG capsules instead, but since we are talking of drinks in this chapter we are focusing in on the green tea itself.

Many integrative physicians use even stronger herbal teas for attacking cancer, such as the South American Taheebo (Pau d'arco) tea that is said to have miraculous healing powers for cancer patients. While it is a tea that you should consider adding to your list of supplemental aids, and while there are many other helpful teas as well, probably the most popular cancer-fighting tea is the famous "Ojibwa tea." This herbal tea remedy originates from the Ojibwa Indians of Canada, who traditionally used it to cure cancer. This famous drink, which is now known as "Essiac tea," is commonly used as an adjunctive to cancer therapies because of its well-known cancer fighting abilities. Sometimes it can control the cancer, sometimes it can help eliminate it and sometimes it only helps to relieve cancer pain. It is commonly used throughout the world by cancer sufferers who want extra help in beating the disease.

This herbal remedy was originally introduced to the general public by Canadian nurse, Rene Caisse, who achieved renown by successfully treating thousands of cancer patients using the Ojibwa formula. The colorful story of the tea has been the subject matter of many books and articles. For instance, the Royal Cancer Commission of Canada held hearings in the 1930's and came to the conclusion that Essiac tea was a cure for cancer. Dr. John Wolfer, director of the tumor clinic at Northwestern University Medical School, arranged for Rene to treat 30 terminal cancer patients under the direction of five physicians. After supervising Essiac therapy for one and a half years, the doctors also concluded that the herbal mixture "prolonged life, shrank tumors, and relieved pain."

In 1937, Dr. Emma Carson spent a month inspecting the Bracebridge Clinic in Canada, where Caisse had worked, and reviewed 400 cases of cancer patients who had been treated with Essiac. In *Options: The Alternative Cancer Therapy Book*, author Richard Walters reports that she said, "The vast majority of Miss Caisse's patients are brought to her for treatment after [conventional treatment] has failed and the patients are pronounced incurable. The actual results from Essiac treatments and the rapidity of repair were absolutely marvelous and must be seen to convincingly confirm belief."

Dr. Charles Brusch, who was the personal physician to President John F. Kennedy, also treated thousands of cancer patients using the Essiac formula. Dr. Brusch stated, "Essiac is a cure for cancer, period." He even used it to cure his own cancer but was placed under a "gag-order" by the Federal Government to not speak about it. His treatment records are still preserved, but as to Rene Caisse's successful treatment records, however, we have an entirely different story.

Immediately upon her death the Canadian Department of National Health and Welfare, for some inexplicable reason, felt compelled to go to her house and burn all her research and records in a 55-gallon oil drum just outside her home. This was not the first unusual thing the government did involving the tea. When the Canadian government had previously found out that sheep sorrel was a major ingredient in the tea, it also immediately banned the sale and distribution of the herb. Strange.

Many books have been written about the properties of Essiac tea (see *Calling of an Angel* by Dr. Gary Glum) and they include many case studies on its powerful cancer fighting abilities. The formula contains herbs with tumor fighting abilities and liver detoxification properties, which is important because you want to be detoxifying your blood and liver when trying to eliminate cancer.

The liver is the major organ in the body that deals with eliminating toxins, and two of the herbs in the formula help protect the liver so that it can better do its job. A person on any cancer treatment releases a lot of toxins into the blood stream, which end up in the liver to be detoxified. As cancer progresses, the damage to the liver usually progresses, too, so any extra detoxification help it gets is a great boost to the body. This is a reason that cancer patients often use coffee enemas.

While it has powerful anti-cancer properties (its cytotoxic effects are only against cancerous cells but not normal healthy cells) and usually makes people feel better, in many cases Essiac/Ojibwa tea is not powerful enough to produce a full cancer recovery alone, which is why it is only considered a supplemental, adjunctive therapy rather than "cancer cure." Once again: *it is not a cure*, so do not depend upon it alone. However, thousands of people have safely used it along with other anti-cancer therapies that their doctors have ordered, so information on Essiac tea is very easy to find due to this great popularity.

Essiac tea is extremely compatible with many types of cancer treatments including chemotherapy, and people often drink 2 ounces three times a day. It may certainly help, and at worst would simply be a waste of money, so you may care to consider using it. Caisse herself felt that while it might not actually cure cancer, it still might offer significant relief.

There are two versions of the tea with different formulas, but both versions seem to have curative effects. The simpler formula seems to be the most preferred. The basic Essiac formula is composed of four immune stimulant, anti-inflammatory, detoxifying and cancer fighting herbs: sheep sorrel, burdock root, slippery elm bark and turkey rhubarb root. Sheep sorrel and burdock root are known to kill cancer cells, and it is of interest that burdock root is also part of the famous Hoxsey herbal cancer cure.

A second formula, available in a bottled version of Essiac, called "Flor-Essence," contains four additional herbs that may or *may not be* part of the original formula: blessed thistle, red clover, watercress and kelp. This eight ingredient herbal concentrate can be purchased at many health food stores and on the internet, but many people do not believe this is the original Essiac formula and therefore do not recommend it.

Many herbalists produce and supply the original Essiac herbal formula for people to brew on their own. This is the one typically preferred. For instance, Essiac-tea.org and Ojibwa Tea of Life (Ojibwatea.com) sell an Ojibwa tea blend comparable to Rene Caisse's original four-herb blend. PlantCures.com sells a similar four-herb blend whose proportions come directly from the Ojibwa Indians. When preparing any formulas, avoid using plastic and aluminum.

All the different versions of Essiac tea seem to have curative effects. However, you must remember that when Rene Caisse used Essiac tea on cancer patients, most of her success came from using an injectable form of the herbs. However, she would make tea that patients would take within 48 hours, whereas tea purchased from stores may be several months old. A problem in some versions is the low quality of the sheep sorrel, which the Canadian government immediately banned for sale after the Essiac formula became known.

Rene Caisse said that sometimes tumors continued to grow larger and harden before breaking down when the tea was being used, which happens during many types of cancer treatment, so warnings are in order for those who have brain tumors, lung cancer, bile duct cancer, cancer of the digestive tract or tumors threatening any major blood supply for the body.

When cancerous tumors are wrapped around an artery, for instance, one has to be careful of all cancer treatments since they typically cause temporary inflammation, swelling and congestion. Inflammation arises when the immune system starts attacking cancer cells as they are dying, which then creates the temporary swelling. Swelling is a sign that the immune system is working hard; however, that same swelling and inflammation can cause partial blockages of fluids or other problems within the body.

Whenever there is a life-threatening blockage due to cancer you should seek medical help immediately. One should therefore check with an integrative cancer specialist as to whether Essiac tea is a complementary fit to one's other cancer therapies. It is rarely used by individuals with kidney problems because two of its herbal ingredients are contraindicated for such cases. This little tidbit of information illustrates the rule to consult an expert before using any of these protocols by yourself or go to a clinic where they are used.

Along these lines, you should remember that organic sulfur protocols can often help cancer patients with the dangers of inflammation and swelling. This is another reason why integrative physicians often combine organic sulfur (MSM/DMSO) with vitamin C (sodium ascorbate rather than citric acid) in protocols that build up the usage gradually over 3-4 days. Together these two substances also help deal with any lactic acid buildup in the body. A final dosage is usually at least 10 grams of MSM and 10 grams of vitamin C per day.

Cesium chloride and DMSO protocols are also used by integrative physicians who want to quickly shrink tumors starting in as little as two weeks. The vitamin C and B12 treatment of Sister Mary Eymard Poydock Ph.D., developed after decades of research, is also said to shrink tumors quickly.

Essiac tea is readily available for purchase on the internet. You can also find out more about the Essiac story from the following publications:

Calling of an Angel, Dr. Gary Glum.

The Essiac Handbook, James Percival.

The Essiac Report: The True Story of a Canadian Herbal Cancer Remedy and of the Thousands of Lives It Continues to Save, Richard Thomas.

Essiac Essentials: The Remarkable Herbal Cancer Fighter, Sheila Snow and Mali Klein.

Essiac: A Native Herbal Cancer Remedy, Cynthia Olsen.

8
LIMU JUICE

Advanced stage cancer patients often need to "buy more time" so that any other therapies they are using have a chance to work. If a cancer therapy normally takes several months to work but you are given fewer months to live, you need something to give you strength and extend your life so that you have time for other cures to become effective.

The most common and logical integrative strategy to extend your life is to supply the normal non-cancerous cells of your body with nutrients (other than sugar) in order to support them. Many people therefore turn to various energizing nutritional powders and/or juices (ex. Boku Superfood, Vitamineral Green, Pure Synergy, grape juice, noni juice, wolfberry juice, mangosteen juice, etc.) for this healthy nourishment. Juices and supergreen powders are an excellent way for cancer patients to absorb huge amounts of nutrition, where they don't have to spend energy digesting it, but can assimilate it rather easily.

Limu juice, which is manufactured from the Limu Moui variety of brown seaweed found in the coastal waters of Tonga, not only does this but also helps to safely kill cancer cells because it contains an active ingredient called "fucoidan." The active cancer-fighting properties of fucoidan are well proven and have appeared in over 100 scientific studies, including Japanese studies showing that seaweeds containing fucoidan caused cancer cell lines to self-destruct. Fucoidan has been found to slow tumor growth, inhibit malignant cancer cells and cause apoptosis. It has no side effects but safely kills cancer cells without harming non-cancerous cells.

In other words, Limu juice, which is made from brown seaweed, both gives your body energy and contains an active cancer-fighting ingredient (fucoidan) that quickly and safely kills cancer cells. Fucoidan is also the main ingredient in **Modifilan**, which is another seaweed extract often used by complementary physicians to help chelate heavy metals from the body to rid it of toxic substances. If you have cancer and need/want to detoxify your body, this is one of the supplements to use.

Many natural substances, like fucoidan, are known to shrink tumors and/or kill cancer cells. Another famous example is laetrile, also known as vitamin B17. *Aloe aborescens* also has active components that fight cancer, as do Graviola and Paw Paw (which are synergistic with chemotherapy), oleander and *nigella sativa* (black cumin). Carrot juice is also known for its compounds that can kill cancer cells. Freshly cut wheatgrass juice has been curing cancer cases for decades because of its constituent ingredients (it is the basis of the Anne Wigmore cancer regimen), and raspberries contain phytonutrients (such as ellagic acid) that have been proven to combat certain types of cancers, too. Purple grapes, which are the basis of the Brandt cancer cure diet, also have nearly a dozen molecules that can kill cancer cells.

As seen, many natural fruits and vegetables are very high in anti-cancer nutrients. Why shouldn't you add them to your diet if you would normally eat them and they certainly don't interfere with mainstream cancer protocols and therapies?

By drinking these particularly helpful fruit and vegetable juices, you will satiate your hunger and crowd out many of the bad foods/drinks from your diet that most people normally consume. You will be consuming a concentrated form of nutrition, which your body can easily absorb without using too much digestive energy. Whilst energizing your body with these highly absorbable nutrients, you will also be providing it with many natural ingredients that fight cancer. I am a firm believer that any cancer patient should be drinking fresh vegetable juices, supplemented with supergreen powders (or turned into green smoothies), several times per day because this will definitely help them to bear traditional treatments or get well.

What is unsafe or illogical about this plan of attack?

While it is not necessary to refrain from all other drinks other than vegetable juices when fighting cancer, complementary physicians often recommend that a cancer patient should attempt to take about 40 ounces of vegetable juices daily to help get well, even if they are not following any anti-cancer juicing protocol, such as the Gerson therapy diet. Even if you cannot drink this amount, drinking some juice is better than drinking none because of the possible benefits.

Limu juice is one of the juices you should especially consider drinking when you have cancer.

Probably the best Limu juice is made from 83% pure Tongan Limu Moui (brown seaweed) and is manufactured by the company that owns the patents for extracting the fucoidan. Since people usually don't like the taste of seaweed by itself, various vendors usually mix Limu juice with other fruit and vegetable juices such as organic papaya, mango, pear, or apple juice, which mask the taste of the seaweed. This makes it much more palatable to drink. Sometimes other botanicals and vitamins are also added to Limu juice by the various juice vendors.

It comes down to this. What should you drink when you have cancer? You already know to stay away from alcohol and sugary beverages, so you must avoid sodas, milk, wine and beer. You should drink clean water free of chlorine and fluoride. There is also green tea and Essiac tea you can drink, and Pau d'arco tea. Pau d'arco tea is another powerful immune-stimulating drink, also known as Taheebo tea (see "Taheebo Life Tea") or Lapacho tea. Many people drink a lot of carrot juice (2-3 times per day) and other special fruits and vegetables when they are on special anti-cancer juicing diets, and now you know about Limu juice, which can be easily purchased through the internet.

Why is this juice cited by itself? Because Limu juice, just by itself, has cured many cancer patients. That's how powerful it is. Thus, it is often used as a stand-alone natural therapy for cancer, since the protocol only entails drinking a tasty beverage, but I would never rely on just this alone. It should always be used as apart of a larger protocol that addresses cancer on many different fronts. In any case, it doesn't interfere with any other prescribed therapies, so why would a physician object?

You should consider adding Limu juice to other effective therapies as an adjunctive supplemental aid, especially for advanced cancer patients. The basic principle is to always use several synergistic cancer protocols at the same time to maximize your odds of eliminating it, and drinking Limu juice is one of the protocols you should consider because its *modus operandi* (involving fucoidan) is different than that of other therapies.

A complementary, integrative physician will always combine various treatments that work on different principles for dealing with cancer. Since cancer's causes are multi-factorial, its treatment should integrate different therapeutic approaches, too, such as boosting the immune system, lowering the microbial load within the body so that the immune system is not distracted, strengthening healthy cells, weakening or destroying cancer cells, alkalizing the body, oxygenating the body, detoxifying the body and trying to revert cancer cells back to normal cells.

Despite its effectiveness, as with all these supplemental aids, you should not consider Limu juice as a cure. It is just another adjunctive cancer treatment aid; a supplemental drink that might help cancer patients gain some time so that their other therapies have a chance to work. It may help extend the life of a patient by several months, which would allow other treatment therapies a chance to do their job. So you might drink Essiac tea, green tea, Lapacho tea, Meso-SGPS or Limu juice, or any combination of these liquids, for all the benefits they might provide.

The minimum amount of Limu juice to drink, for any beneficial therapeutic effect, is 16 ounces a day for an adult. This daily minimum dose of 16 ounces should be spread out among several small glasses to be taken throughout the day. Furthermore, some have stated that Limu Juice should not be taken for 48 hours after a chemotherapy treatment in order to allow the chemo to do its work. Naturally, as with all these supplemental aids, you should check these instructions with your physician.

The many beneficial cancer-fighting properties of fucoidan are easily researched on the web and you can find out more about Limu Moui by reading:

Limu Moui: Prize Sea Plant of the South Pacific, Rita Elkins.

9
ALOE ARBORESCENS

Several books have been written about the Brazilian *Aloe aborescens* cancer protocol and the fascinating story about how a Franciscan Friar, Father Romano Zago, discovered this all-natural recipe being used to cure cancer in the slums of Brazil. Since that time, Father Zago has made it part of his life mission to popularize this simple, natural remedy.

For some people the *Aloe aborescens* formula has cured their cancer just by itself and for others not, which is why it is considered a supplemental rather than a standalone helpmate, like all these therapies being revealed. This therapy is so simple that it can be readily added to any list of complementary therapies. While it has been used as the singular stand-alone "cancer cure" in the slums of Brazil and has over 1,000 testimonials to its credit, wisdom suggests it be used as a supplemental protocol, together with other effective cancer treatments, so that the combination of synergistic approaches becomes more powerful than using just one approach alone.

Aloe arborescens, which is at the heart of the protocol, is basically a special species of aloe (called "Torch aloe" because of the plant's bright red flowers) that has special anti-inflammatory and immunomodulation properties. It has about twice the number of active medicinal ingredients as the ordinary *Aloe vera* plant. Even still, *Aloe vera* contains a rich content of polysaccharide glyconutrients that are potent immune system stimulators and is often used itself in various naturopathic cancer protocols.

The Brazilian *Aloe arborescens* cancer protocol is extremely simple. Each day you drink three tablespoons of a mixture of three ingredients: *Aloe arborescens*, alcohol and honey. The aloe contains the active ingredients that fight cancer. The alcohol enlarges a patient's blood vessels to help deliver the formula ingredients. The raw honey (which contains glucose sugar) helps transport the aloe-nutrients into the cells, like a Trojan horse, so that they can be destroyed. This is the same strategy as therapies that use DMSO to open the pores of cancer cells, so that more cancer-fighting ingredients can get into the cells.

Here is how the "Trojan horse" strategy works. Cancer cells are almost entirely dependent on glucose for survival. They have up to 15 times more insulin receptors than normal cells so that they can greedily absorb glucose from the bloodstream. Because a cancer cell has more insulin receptors than normal cells, we can feed the body glucose that will then cause a cancer cell to greedily open up its pores for this food, at which time it will readily accept other substances and draw them into the cell.

This is also the strategy oncologists use with Insulin Potentiation Theory to feed cancerous tumors the toxic chemicals of chemotherapy. Basically, one can kill a cancerous cell with much lower doses of chemotherapy using this mechanism. So just as glucose is used to efficiently carry radiological materials into sugar loving cancer cells for PET scans, the glucose from the honey is used to carry the active *Aloe arborescens* ingredients into the cancer cells, where they can begin to attack the cancer. The honey also helps to balance the slightly bitter taste of the aloe.

As stated, the *Aloe aborescens* drink is typically used as a supplemental aid for cancer treatments and is often used in conjunction with chemotherapy because it is said to significantly reduce chemotherapy side effects. Although it is used to fight cancer, it can also be used as a cancer preventative, as a remission protocol and also for radiation burns.

The basic formula, which you are not advised to prepare on your own because of possible errors, is made according to the following recipe. You take roughly equal amounts of unpasteurized raw honey and the 5-year old leaves of *Aloe aborescens* and mix them with a 1% alcohol distillate. To prepare the mixture, you remove the spines of the aloe leaves and place the three ingredients in a blender, blending them well to obtain a light mixture.

You must process the mixture without heating, cold pressing or freeze drying. The ingredients:

- About half a kilogram (about 18 ounces, or 1.1 pounds) of raw bee's honey (not refined or synthetic honey)
- 2 *Aloe arborescens* leaves
- 3-4 spoonfuls of alcohol distillate (such as brandy, cognac or whisky) to preserve the product and dilate the blood vessels so the treatment can reach all parts of the body.

Father Zago's usage instructions are as follows. A person takes one dose, three times a day (i.e. three tablespoons a day) before breakfast, lunch and dinner. The doses are taken on an empty stomach 10 to 30 minutes before a meal, and nothing else is taken afterwards until 20 or 30 minutes have gone by. One should shake the mixture very well just before pouring out the tablespoon to be ingested.

The recipe should be taken 10 days on, 10 days off, 10 days on, 10 days off, etc. in repeating cycles. However, a person can also take this protocol without any "days off" if they so desire. Zago's book also says that if you have taken the protocol of 10 days on and 10 days off for four repetitions, and you have still not achieved your objective, then you should double the dose until you meet your objective. This is the problem with it in that it often requires a long time to produce healing.

Father Zago also advises that a cancer patient should stop the protocol entirely only after they have regained their strength and feel their cancer is in complete remission. He has emphasized that it is extremely important that a cancer patient does not stop using this protocol until there is complete remission, otherwise prematurely stopping the use of the protocol will allow the cancer to come back. For someone who is in remission, the formula should still be used (in the normal 10 days on, 10 days off cycle) every three months for at least two years after the patient is declared to be in remission.

It is very difficult to make this product correctly at home because it requires the exact species, *Aloe aborescens*, and one must use the older (and hard to find) leaves of a plant that is at least 5 years old. It is also difficult to process *Aloe aborescens* correctly to maintain its cancer fighting properties. There are many important rules about when to cut the leaves, how to process them and other details that can be found in Zago's two books, if you wish to do this. The simpler and better way than trying to make the product on your own (and risk an incorrect/useless preparation) is to buy an already prepared mixture that was properly produced according to the correct instructions.

Once made or purchased, the *Aloe arborescens* mixture should be stored in a cool, dark place away from light. If you store it in a refrigerator, you should even keep the bottle inside of a dark container (or cover it with a dark sock) to shield it from the light exposure of the refrigerator door being opened many times a day. As stated, the product should *never* come into direct contact with sunlight, which makes this a somewhat fragile therapy. Even when ingesting the product you should avoid any type of light exposure as much as possible. For instance, after you pour the product into the tablespoon you should immediately drink it to allow as little contact time with light as possible. A brief explanation for this is that sunlight contains ultraviolet radiation, which can alter chemically alter active molecules in the preparation.

This treatment will start to cleanse your body because most aloe plants are detoxifiers, so it is normal to experience various detoxification reactions after starting to use it. This includes the possibility of loose stools or skin rashes for the first few days, as it starts to detoxify the blood. As with any protocol that deals with toxins, there may be some uncomfortable reactions to the formula that include a wide range of typical detox symptoms, but none of these are serious.

Information on the *Aloe arborscens* protocol is readily found on the internet. You can also find out more about this protocol from the following publications:

Cancer Can Be Cured!, OFM Romano Zago.

Aloe Isn't Medicine, and Yet ... It Cures, OFM Romano Zago.

Hydrogen Peroxide and Aloe Vera Plus Other Home Remedies, Conrad Lebeau.

Some people who use this formula say that it definitely helped them avoid the terrible side effects of chemotherapy. Reliable sources for a correctly prepared product having the correct ingredients with the right proportions include:

Quantum Nutrition, Austin, Texas 888-588-7590 (USA)
Aloeproductscenter.com
Quantumnutrition.com
Aloearborescens.org/products
Aloeone.co.uk (UK)
Aloedipadreromanozago.it (Italy)

10
LOW DOSE NALTREXONE

One of the special pharmaceutical substances originally used to fight HIV/AIDs, which has also been found to do a wonderful job with cancer, is low-dose naltrexone (LDN). "Naltrexone" is the chemical name of this pharmaceutical, but Dupont sells it under the brand name of "ReVia," Mallinckrodt as "Depade" and Barr Laboratories sells it under the generic name "naltrexone."

Naltrexone is a powerful immune modulator, and its use for cancer is a powerful but extremely effective "off label" use of the medication. Since low-dose naltrexone therapy involves taking just one tiny pill at night, it may be one of the easiest cancer treatments ever developed, and it is extremely inexpensive, too.

You will have to ask your doctor for a prescription to follow this highly effective therapy, just as you must if you wanted to use Dr. Robert Jones' highly successful but inexpensive do-it-yourself Phenergan protocol as a cancer treatment. However, because LDN therapy is so simple and only requires swallowing a single small pill every night before bedtime, it is being included because of its power and simplicity. LDN therapy makes some patients feel dramatically better within days.

In *Defeat Cancer; 15 Doctors of Integrative and Naturopathic Medicine Tell You How* (Connie Strasheim), Dr. Elio M. Rivera Celaya is reported to have said, "This one compound, by itself, is more powerful and effective for treating cancer than almost anything in the conventional treatment arsenal." In the same book, Dr. Martin Dayton reported yet another of the miraculous cases of patients who responded wonderfully to low-dose naltrexone tablets. Many physicians have proven its benefits on a wide variety of autoimmune conditions and its efficacy and safety has been demonstrated in thousands of cases. It is a non-toxic treatment without any side effects and can even be used during chemotherapy.

So what exactly does naltrexone do?

At an extremely low dose of approximately 4.5 mg once a day, taken at bedtime (between 9 pm and 3 am), naltrexone boosts the body's immune system by increasing natural killer cells and other healthy immune defenses against cancer and it reduces inflammation. It is thought that it also works on the opioid receptors of cancer cells as an anti-growth factor and perhaps, induces cancer cell death (apoptosis). While its means of operation is still under research, it definitely activates the body's own natural defenses to greatly benefit cancer patients. This is a different approach than the traditional trio of surgery, chemo or radiation.

The effectiveness of low-dose naltrexone (LDN) for cancer patients was first discovered by Dr. Bernard Bihari in the mid-1990's. Dr. Bihari found that his cancer patients were greatly helped, in some cases dramatically, from just a small amount of the pharmaceutical. When used for HIV, LDN radically increases natural killer cell activity and is 95% effective in stopping the progression of HIV to AIDS. It eliminates opportunistic infections (which also often plague cancer patients undergoing various mainstream therapies) and can make people well enough to hold full-time jobs.

Dr. Bihari has used low-dose naltrexone on hundreds of cancer patients, almost all of whom had failed to respond to standard, conventional treatments such as chemotherapy. His results suggest that more than 60% of cancer patients may significantly benefit from LDN in seeing a stabilization of their condition, major tumor shrinkage or a move toward total remission.

With conventional cancer treatments, usually a patient either dies or is totally cured whereas with LDN therapy, a third alternative becomes possible that is revolutionary for the cancer industry: the long-term stabilization and/or gradual reduction of the size of a tumor so that cancer can, in some cases, simply become a manageable chronic disease like diabetes. By itself, LDN therapy gives some cancer patients the possibility of living free of symptoms, without them having to suffer the crippling side effects of chemotherapy or radiation treatment.

While Dr. Bihari has achieved impressive results with his usage of low-dose naltrexone for cancer patients, LDN therapy has not undergone a full blown clinical trial. Nevertheless, the many doctors who have used it swear by its effectiveness and it is backed by many years of published, supportive laboratory research findings. For instance, laboratory research studies by I. Zagon, Ph.D. have over many years demonstrated the inhibition of a number of different human tumors by low-dose naltrexone.

Naltrexone can only be obtained through a doctor's prescription, so your physician would have to prescribe it after deciding it is right for you. It is extremely inexpensive (less than $20/month) and a prescription can be fulfilled by hundreds of local pharmacies. The typical therapeutic dosage is 1.5 mg to 4.5 mg, and it should *not* be provided in slow-release or time-release form. There are special usage instructions for those taking thyroid replacement hormones, patients who have undergone organ replacements, and for those on narcotic medications like morphine, since it blocks opioid receptors within the body for 3-4 hours.

Since it is harmless but might greatly help, there is no reason to fear LDN. A cancer patient can safely consider LDN while on chemotherapy or post-treatment, to prevent a recurrence of tumors. LDN has even been shown to work with virtually incurable cancers such as multiple myeloma, neuroblastoma and pancreatic cancer. It is an effective treatment for many types of disease other than just cancer, simply because it stimulates the immune system.

You can find full details of the usage of low-dose naltrexone and countless medical studies on its usage at Lowdosenaltrexone.org or Ldninfo.org. Another book that discusses the proper usage of LDN is:

Immune Restoration Handbook, Conrad LeBeau.

11
OLEANDER EXTRACT

In 1966 a Turkish doctor, Dr. Huseyin Zima Ozel, was searching for a cancer remedy when he discovered a group of rural villagers who were amazingly healthy compared to other similar villagers in Turkey. Upon investigation, he found that these healthy villagers were all taking a 2000-year old folk remedy that was based on a common plant, referred to in the Bible as the "Desert Rose," namely the oleander plant (*Nerium oleander*).

The oleander plant is highly toxic in raw form, but a wonderful remedy for immune conditions when properly prepared. It contains over 500 compounds, many of which have been noted for their cancer fighting or immune stimulating abilities. It is a strong immune booster that contains molecules that can cross the blood-brain barrier, inhibit angiogenesis, inhibit the ability of cancer cells to defend themselves when they come under attack, and induce apoptosis (normal cell death) in cancer cells. Basically, it fights cancer in multiple ways.

After his discovery that *Nerium oleander* could be used to treat cancer, Dr. Ozel (Drozel.com) started making a medicine out of it that he used as a cancer treatment for over 40 years. He patented an aqueous extract of oleander, whose trademark name is "Anvirzel," which has a reported success rate of over 70%. There are many case studies available on oleander extract, such as a successful double-blind trial in South Africa that showed it to be successful in stabilizing and reversing HIV symptoms, and useful against a wide variety of cancers.

Oleander has been very successful in human use, but this therapy works very slowly. You are unlikely to see major results within a short period of two months, but during that time it typically starts to slow tumor growth. Oleander can be used alone or with other immune-boosting supplements, and even with prescription medications or chemotherapy and radiation treatments (though of course you must check with your doctor). For the best results, it should always be taken within a broader immune-boosting anti-cancer protocol, since this will maximize its effectiveness. It is said to be highly compatible with the Budwig diet.

When you use chemo or radiation and add oleander extract to your protocol, it is reported to either eliminate or greatly reduce virtually all of the side effects associated with such treatments, including hair loss (except with cisplatin). Oleander typically potentiates chemotherapy and radiation when used as a complementary therapy. Unlike chemotherapy, however, oleander usually increases a cancer patient's energy levels.

Oleander can be prepared in a soup, but because of its toxicity this is considered more dangerous than using an oleander extract because the toxic oils of the plant are removed during manufacturing to prepare extract concentrates. No reports of toxicity have ever been received by the many clinicians using oleander extract therapy. However, if you are worried about toxicity then this is a supplemental therapy to avoid.

A popular oleander extract, named "Sutherlandia OPC," has been used for many years in South Africa to treat HIV and cancer (see Sutherlandiaopc.com). It is a combination of the Turkish folk remedy *Nerium Oleander*, which, as stated, has been used for thousands of years, and the local *Sutherlandia Fructescens* (South African "Cancer Bush"). Thousands of people have now used this remedy for cancer and other immune conditions over the past several years and there has not been a single report of a serious adverse reaction or side effect.

A newer version of oleander extract, called "Rose Laurel OPC Plus," also made by the manufacturer of Sutherlandia OPC, is now available for purchase from the Utopia Silver Supplements company (Utopiasilver.com). The new version contains only oleander extract powder and has 33% more oleander than the original Sutherlandia OPC. As with the original product, there haven't been any reports of serious adverse reactions or side effects for the extract taken according to directions.

This new formulation is now the most common oleander product of choice for cancer patients, especially more advanced, aggressive and/or difficult cancer cases. It is usually used in conjunction with the complementary supplement N-Acetyl-Cysteine (NAC) to help prevent cachexia. Remember that to help prevent cachexia you need to consume enough protein, otherwise cancer cells will start consuming your body to get it. A systemic review of 17 studies on omega-3 fatty acids found evidence that they would benefit cancer patients in many ways, one of which was by specifically preventing cachexia. Hence the goal of preventing cachexia is yet another reason to consider adding the Budwig FOCC mixture to your diet since it contains these fatty acids.

The suggested dosage for either the Rose Laurel OPC Plus or Sutherandia OPC supplement are the same: instructions normally call for 5 to 25 ml of extract three times daily, or 3 to 9 capsules daily in divided doses, taken with meals. The number of doses (size of dosage) depends on the weight of the patient and stage and aggressiveness of the cancer. For calculation purposes, one teaspoon of liquid extract (5 ml) is equivalent to about 1 capsule of extract. The liquid extract, rather than the capsules, is often used in cases of rectal or liver cancer, when there are malabsorption problems due to problems with the stomach or intestines.

Why does oleander work? It is thought that its efficacy is due to its combined active ingredients rather than just one single compound. A departmental head at the MD Anderson Cancer Center in Houston is reported to have said, "We don't know yet exactly how it works, we just know that it does work, attacking and killing bad cells - and only bad cells - and stopping their multiplication." Oleander extract is basically a substance that attacks cancer directly, but since oleander does not protect healthy normal cells, when using it you would also want to support your healthy cells and immune system through various other nutritional protocols. This knocks out its consideration as a top strategy of choice.

Remember, oleander is very toxic in its raw form but the version discussed is medicinal oleander extract. As with all these natural supplements, you should definitely clear the usage of this product with your doctor, in particular if you are taking blood thinner medications (since it helps to thin the blood), or if you are on heart drugs, such as anti-arrhythmics.

Various forum groups on the internet discuss the use of oleander for cancer (Oleandersoup.com). The websites Tbyil.com, Curezone.com and Cancertutor.com can also be referenced for more valuable information on oleander extract therapy, as well as the book:

Cancer's Natural Enemy, Tony Isaacs.

12

DR. MATTHIAS RATH'S
ANTI-METASTASIS FORMULA

Many discoveries in the medical field are often overlooked or suppressed for various reasons. For instance, Sister Mary Eymard Poydock Ph.D., director of cancer research at Mereyhurst College in Erie, Pennsylvania, worked for twenty years to develop a means of inhibiting cancer growth by injecting a combination of vitamin C and vitamin B12 near a tumor site. When the two vitamins are injected in a ratio of one part vitamin B12 to one part vitamin C, it can stop tumor cell growth entirely. Sometimes tumors can disappear within days, which makes this an interesting option when a doctor suggests a mastectomy to remove a lump. Many other natural substances also destroy tumors when injected into them.

After developing her tumor shrinking anti-growth approach for decades, Sister Poydock stated, "We've got it down to a point now where, if you do it according to the 'recipe,' it will work every time." Unfortunately, like our next protocol, medical science seems to have ignored her approach despite its excellent results and all her published research.

Her approach introduces a major concern for cancer patients called metastasis, which is the invasive spread of cancer to other areas of the body. With metastasis, cancer cells secrete millions of enzyme molecules that act like little scissors. These enzymes cut the collagen connective tissue that surrounds cells, and they cut holes in the walls of blood vessels. This then enables the cancer cells to get into the blood stream and migrate to other areas, where they then settle and start new tumor growth (secondary cancers). This needs to be prevented.

The medical approach of using specific pharmaceutical drugs to contain metastasis has not been hugely successful in modern medicine. Even current treatment protocols that involve chemotherapy or radiation focus on cancer cell destruction, but they do not address the problem of metastasis. In short, *there are not really any conventional medical means available to control cancer metastasis.*

Luckily German physician Dr. Matthias Rath, who worked with two-time Nobel Prize winner Linus Pauling (who lived with full vitality until age 96 by taking large daily doses of vitamin C, thus far outliving all of his naysaying detractors), developed a very simple combination of amino acids to help prevent metastasis. It is a proven formula often used by integrative physicians worried about the spread of cancer throughout the body.

The story behind the development of this natural, non-toxic protocol is as follows.

Many years ago, Linus Pauling and his associate, Dr. Ewan Cameron, performed a study which unmistakably proved that an intravenous vitamin C dosage of 10 grams a day given to terminal cancer patients could extend their life expectancy by a factor of five times or more. This simple vitamin C protocol does not "cure cancer," but it definitely extends human life by protecting non-cancerous cells. This is why intravenous vitamin C therapy is used by many integrative physicians. By extending a patient's life with this simple technique, other cancer treatments *may then have five times as long to work at becoming effective.* Think about this! It "buys time" for a patient so that other treatment therapies, mainstream or not, have a chance to work, which is why so many integrative physicians use this regimen.

Perhaps the reason vitamin C works so well against cancer is because the vitamin C molecule looks so similar to glucose. Cancer cells actively take in more glucose than normal cells, and thus they may transport high levels of vitamin C into themselves simply because of the similar shape.

Once inside the cancer cell, high levels of vitamin C will react with intracellular iron and copper to produce small amounts of hydrogen peroxide, which will eventually build up to a concentration strong enough that it will lyse (dissolve or destroy) the cancer cell from inside. This would explain why high doses of intravenous vitamin C works so selectively against cancer cells and not normal cells. Linus Pauling and Dr. Ewan Cameron were able to extend the lives of cancer patients just from this simple therapy alone.

However, modern integrative oncologists have improved upon this approach by adding DMSO to this therapy since it helps to open up the cancer cell ports that make it even easier for vitamin C to enter the cells. In 1968 it was proven that DMSO has an affinity for cancer cells, and is absorbed into tumors instead of healthy cells. DMSO can bind to various substances and drag them into cancer cells, including the chemicals agents used by mainstream chemotherapy (see Ross Hauser's *Treating Cancer with Insulin Potentiation Therapy*). It has even been shown to help cancer cells *revert to normal cells* (see John Boik's *Cancer & Natural Medicine: A Textbook of Basic Science and Clinical Research*). In any case, it allows even more vitamin C to enter cancer cells than what would normally be absorbed into those cells. When you simultaneously go on a low glucose diet, this is even more reason for the hungry cancer cells, looking for food, to greedily absorb the vitamin C into themselves.

If you think about it, you can realize that vitamin C can help a cancer patient in many additional ways, too. It will boost your immune system function because it will energize white blood cells. It may work to kill any microbes within the body that may play a role in causing cancer. It will induce cancer cells to die early, so it will directly help to kill cancer cells. It can also stimulate collagen formation to help the body wall off a tumor.

Having worked with Linus Pauling and being very familiar with his work, in 1991 Dr. Matthias Rath found that the amino acid lysine, when combined with vitamin C, inhibited the action of protease in the body. Protease is an enzyme secreted by cancer cells to digest collagen within the body, which is necessary for cancer to spread to areas far away. Thus, using vitamin C and lysine at the same time allows them to work together to help isolate cancer cells by preventing collagen destruction, which helps to then prevent cancer cells from spreading.

In 2002, Rath and other researchers discovered that adding the amino acid proline and EGCG (our previously mentioned anti-cancer agent found in green tea) to this basic protocol *stopped* the protease destruction of collagen connective tissue. Vitamin C, lysine and proline are necessary components for the production of collagen and elastin within the body. They are responsible for building strong connective tissue within us. When you supply them to a cancer patient, along with EGCG, the total combination helps stop the destruction of this connective tissue by cancer.

Vitamin C and lysine are not normally produced in the human body, so you need to get them from the diet. The idea of their supplementation in cancer cases to build stronger connective tissue becomes logical when you realize what they do and that many people are nutritionally deficient. By supplementing with substances that will increase the strength of the connective tissue surrounding cancer cells, this will help to encapsulate the tumor and prevent metastasis.

The "Dr. Rath Cellular Solution" for inhibiting cancer metastasis therefore is an entirely natural anti-cancer formula consisting of l-lysine and l-proline along with vitamin C and the epigallocatechin gallate (EGCG) found in Green Tea. Laboratory trials and human trials (see the studies below) have proven the effectiveness of this formula (blocking the spread of skin or breast cancer cells in experiments by 100% and 91% respectively) and there are even testimonials that it has cured difficult cases of brain and bone cancer when used in conjunction with a strict diet and other measures.

You should discuss with your physician whether you should add this simple protocol to your cancer treatment plan. This natural regimen does not interfere with chemotherapy or radiation, and in fact the vitamin C reduces the side effects of these treatments and helps with internal healing, while EGCG is known to help potentize the effectiveness of chemotherapy! If you choose to undergo chemotherapy, you should want your healthy cells to be protected (by the vitamin C) and you want the chemo to be more effective (because of the EGCG) while metastasis is inhibited.

The following therapeutic dosages approximate a basic Rath protocol. It can be taken throughout the day in divided doses (or multiple times for a larger net amount) so that the ingredients are steadily delivered to the body:

- L-lysine (~1000 mg)
- L-proline (~750 mg)
- Vitamin C (~700 mg – try to use high grade ascorbic acid powder)
- EGCG (~1000 mg - which can be obtained through capsules and also by drinking green tea; specially powdered Matcha green tea contains a high concentration of EGCG per cup)

This protocol not only inhibits metastasis by preventing the destruction of connective tissue, but helps you quickly regenerate and rebuild any collagen already destroyed by cancer. You don't have to take these as separate supplements, but can find a combination of these ingredients in a product formulated by Rath called "**Epican Forte.**" That makes this easy to use.

Copper also participates along with vitamin C, proline and lysine in the synthesis of collagen and elastin, but Rath did not investigate its participatory role in preserving or building collagen. Some doctors tell cancer patients to avoid copper because it is theoretically implicated in angiogenesis, and therefore they allow patients to suffer copper deficiencies during cancer treatments without considering its many uses elsewhere. However, its possible contribution to inhibiting metastasis through this mechanism needs to be investigated. Recent research on mice showed that various copper complexes would decrease their tumor growths and inhibit metastasis because they helped cancer cells revert to normal cells. Research in France from the 1930's also showed that colloidal copper injections helped to mobilize and expel tumor tissues.

In any case, you can use Epican Forte on your own upon your physician's approval. You can also find out more about Rath's natural anti-metastasis protocol, which is said to have cured brain and bone cancer, by pursuing the following papers that you might wish to share with your doctor:

"A Specific Combination of Ascorbic Acid, Lysine, Proline and Epigallocatechin Gallate Inhibits Proliferation and Extracellular Matrix Invasion of Various Human Cancer Cell Lines." Shriranf P Netke, W Waheed Roomi, Vadim Ivanov, Alekandra Niedzwiecki and Matthias Rath. *Emerging Drugs - Vol. II*, 2003. Author for correspondence and reprints: Matthias Rath, Matthias Rath, Inc., Research and Development, Santa Clara, CA 95054. Phone (408) 807-5564; FAX: (408) 986-9403.

"A Natural Anti-Cancer Formula - A Specific Formulation of Nutrients Containing Lysine, Proline, Ascorbic Acid, and Epigallocatechin Gallate Inhibits Matrix Metalloproteinases Activity and Invasion Potential of Human Cancer Cell Lines." M.W. Roomi, S.P. Netke, V. Ivanov, M. Rath and A. Niedzwiecki. Presented at: European Organization for Research and Treatment of Cancer (EORTC), AACR and NCI Symposium on Molecular Targets and Cancer Therapeutics, Frankfurt, Germany, Nov 19-22, 2002; Published in: European Cancer Journal, 38, Suppl. 7/Abs. 280, 2002.

"Inhibitory Effect of a Natural Anti-Cancer Formula - A Specific Formulation of Nutrients Containing Lysine, Proline, Ascorbic Acid and Epigallocatechin Gallate on the Matrix Metalloproteinases Activities and Invasion of Human Fibrosarcoma HT-1080 Cells." MW Roomi, V Ivanov, SP Netke, M Rath and A Niedzwiecki. *FASEB Journal* (2003) 8452.

"Inhibitory effects of ascorbic acid, proline and lysine supplementation on Matrigel invasion by human breast cancer cells, MDA-MB231." S Netke, Ph.D., V Ivanov , MD. Ph.D., W. Roomi, Ph. D., A Niedzwiecki, Ph. D., Matthias Rath, M.D. Presented at: 19th Annual Miami Breast Cancer Conference, Miami Beach, Florida, February 27 - March 3, 2002. Published in: Conference Proceedings.

"Matrix Metalloproteinase-2 Inhibition and Invasion Potential in Human Chondrocytes by a natural anti-cancer formula - a Specific Mixture of Nutrients Containing Lysine, Proline, Ascorbic Acid and Epigallocatechin Gallate." M.W. Roomi, S.P. Netke, V. Ivanov, M. Rath and A. Niedzwiecki. Presented at: American Association of Cancer Research Special Conference in Cancer Research: Proteases, Extracellular Matrix and Cancer, Hilton Head Island, South Carolina, Oct 9-13, 2002.

OTHER
HELPFUL
AIDS

13
POSITIVE THOUGHTS
AND MEDITATION PRACTICE

Many doctors will tell you that there is a spiritual, emotional and mental component to defeating cancer. They will emphasize that your emotional wellbeing is necessary for healing and that there is a high correlation between beating cancer and breaking any ingrained negative thought patterns. Instead of disrupting emotions, peace in your life will definitely assist your healing.

In other words, your state of mind will definitely influence your ability to beat cancer and survive. The moods of depression, anger or fear will pose barriers to healing and the attitudes of hate, self-righteousness or long suppressed bitterness will hamper healing, too. Practicing the Emotional Freedom Technique (EFT), which involves tuning into a particular problem and reciting healing affirmations while tapping on acupuncture meridians, may help you get rid of many of the negative thoughts and emotions you wish you didn't continually hold onto and which might be blocking healing.

Sometimes an oncologist will suggest a "change of scenery" or other positive activities to help a cancer patient leave an emotional rut. They will tell you to get out of the house and walk in the sunshine (which raise your spirits and increase your vitamin D levels), stay optimistic, laugh more, and even to practice meditation. In some cases they will tell you to learn a craft, pursue some activity you always wanted or take a trip if it will put you into more positive spirits. The basic idea is that you should put your mind on positive, creative things rather than remain preoccupied with worrying, sad or depressing thoughts involved with cancer and the possibility of death.

In short, to beat cancer you should try to make some major changes in your mental attitude. If there is such a thing as emotions activating cancer genes, you need to stop holding onto negative emotions such as hate and start practicing more positive alternatives, such as forgiveness. You must stop holding onto any lingering feelings of ill will towards others. Sometimes holding onto secrets will keep you sick, too. You must also abandon feelings of helplessness and despair to cultivate an optimistic "can do" fighting attitude. Of course the very next step is to take this educational information and find a health expert to help you put it into practice.

Assertive behavior increases cancer survival dramatically, and being assertive includes giving up burdens that have been holding you down, so that you finally feel fully free to express yourself. All these things will help you heal.

Many people take their cancer as a positive "wake up call" to change their life for the better and start doing what really matters to them in life, which is sometimes what they have strictly denied themselves. Along these positive transformations, you must also change your diet and nutrition if you want to feel better while fighting cancer. Anything that finally allows the suppressed energy that's been bottled up inside you to flow throughout your body unfettered is entirely beneficial because it is contributive to healing.

There is a definite tendency for cancer survivors to be positive about their future and get deeply involved in the healing process. They *work their program*; they become committed to following a disciplined regime for a long time. It is typical that many use a multitude of nutraceuticals (such as those presented within this book) and dietary changes rather than just one single thing to get well, and they concentrate on the essential rather than the superficial. Knowing the actual dismal "cure rates" of conventional cancer therapies, they decide to take charge of their own health care, rather than just blindly follow the suggestions of their doctors.

Many cancer survivors choose to work with a cancer expert coach, or depend on other professionals to help guide their recovery and then stay well. Some of the very best protocols and cancer experts in the world are at clinics in Mexico, South America and Germany, so that is where they often head. Whether or not you take this approach, you should try to develop a support network of family and friends to help you with your efforts.

Is there more you can do?

Of course, and one of the things that many integrative oncologists particularly recommend is the practice of meditation.

Previously we mentioned John Boik's book, *Cancer and Natural Medicine*, which has been endorsed by several physicians. It provides all sorts of information on alternative remedies for cancer as well as the actual survival statistics that your doctor is not likely to tell you.

In this book, Boik specifically talks about the practice of meditation and its positive effects on cancer healing. He discusses the findings of Australian psychiatrist, Ainslie Meares, who discovered how cancer patients should best practice meditation in order to go into remission. Meares found that the most effective meditation discipline for cancer patients, of the ones he studied, was a series of intensive sessions of imageless meditation that is typically called "emptiness meditation."

In other words, "emptiness meditation" (which means reaching a mental state where the mind doesn't cling to thoughts and they subsequently calm down) produced the best healing results for cancer, and was the most helpful when people were using meditation in conjunction with modern medicine for cancer treatments. If you think that meditation by itself will cure your cancer or rely upon this notion, you are abandoning common sense and entering a world of false hopes and delusion. It can be a very helpful adjunctive practice, like many of these other supplemental therapies discussed, but is not a "cancer cure."

In a 1976 article published in the *Medical Journal of Australia* ("Regression of Cancer After Intensive Meditation"), Meares found that meditation definitely reduced the anxiety, depression and pain of cancer patients, which is not surprising since it typically does this for any health condition. He also surprisingly reported that approximately 10% of cancer patients achieved remission through this style of meditation practice. In other words, meditation inhibited the growth of tumors in 10% of the cases he studied and improved the quality of life in 50% of cancer cases. It consistently produced significantly longer survival rates and facilitated death with dignity in 90% of the cases studied.

The meditation method Meares taught involves first achieving a state of physical relaxation. The next step is that you should try to empty your mind by letting go of your thoughts, so that you achieve some state of mental quiet where thoughts are relatively absent. You can find several excellent ways to quickly reach this state in *Easy Meditation Lessons* (Bodri & Lee) or *The Little Book of Meditation* (Bodri). Meares commented, "This type of meditation is characterized by extreme simplicity and stillness of the mind, and so differs from other forms of relaxation, meditation or auto-hypnosis that employ the use of a mantra, awareness of your breathing, or mental visualization of the healing process."

There are many parallels here with the common counsel given to cancer patients to let go of any negative thought patterns they have been holding onto (such as thoughts of bitterness, hate and ill will). It is said that clinging to those negative patterns impedes one's internal energy circulation, which acupuncture treatments try to stimulate, and thus stands in the way of healing. When you finally let go of these negative patterns, you will release internal energies that have been bound by restriction so that they are finally freely available for health and healing.

Often you will find that people who hate their jobs or careers get cancer. When they finally just stop and say "the heck with it" to abandon what they have been forcing themselves to miserably endure for decades, they often start to get well. The natural internal energy flow within their bodies, which has been dammed up because they have been suppressing it for so long, can finally assume its natural circulation upon mental release, and with this return to normality cancer often goes into remission.

In other words, if you build for yourself an artificial cocoon of negative thoughts and habits that bind you, while you simultaneously suppress your real interests and desires, this inhibition of your life force will affect your health. By suppressing what is most important to you in life, such as the natural joy for life and your desired avenues of expression, it is possible to become sick. If you let go of that negativity, you have found part of the formula for healing.

Meditation is the one mental practice that helps you to abandon these negative thought patterns that you have created for yourself, so that you can achieve a more normal, natural energy flow within your body that benefits healing. To attain this, Meares taught a method of meditation that was essentially an "effortless stilling of the mind." He discouraged the popular guided visualization-imagery methods proposed by many psychologists today. He found that there were three common characteristics to the meditation practices that produced the most improvements in cancer patients:

- It was profound and prolonged (the "successful" patients practiced at least 20 sessions of intensive meditation)
- It involved little or no conscious activity (which is the definition of "emptiness meditation")
- The practitioners carried the meditation practice of mentally letting go into their daily lives.

While there is a large body of research proving that meditation can produce physiological changes in the human body, if you want to learn any meditation practice at all, you should therefore try to learn some form of emptiness meditation as another adjunctive cancer therapy. This is the type of meditation that can help you get well. You want to learn a meditation technique that helps you quiet your mind and then learn to take that relatively quiet/empty mental state with you into the regular world.

There is a famous meditation you might practice that quickly leads to the "mental emptiness" state that Meares found helpful. It is traditionally used when people get sick, and there is one particular version of this meditation practice that is especially used for cases of cancer.

The instructions for this helpful meditation practice are as follows: You sit quietly, adjust your body and breathing so that they both calm down, and then visualize stripping away all the flesh from your bones, starting from your feet working upwards, until you are just a sitting white skeleton. In other words, after your flesh is gone, you imagine sitting there being just a pure white skeleton – a pure white set of bones. You hold onto that image of just being a bright white skeleton until the image in your mind becomes stable, and then you imagine that your skeleton transforms into dust, which then blows away so that you are left with an infinite mental visage of empty space. Once you reach the stage where everything is just empty space, you just rest in that empty (relatively thoughtless) mental condition, without clinging to any mental thing that arises.

This meditation practice will quickly produce a very quiet, empty mind, which is exactly what Meares found most helpful for cancer patients. When you experience this final stage of mental quiet, you should just let go of everything and stay in that thought-free state for as long as possible. You can achieve this state of "mental emptiness" either by directly letting go of thoughts, or by first focusing on a mental image so that you attain mental stability and then letting go of that state.

Eastern medical teachings explain that the longer you stay there in an empty state of mind, the easier it will be for your internal energy to arise along your acupuncture meridians, to help push sickness out of your body. Acupuncture tries to stimulate this energy through a purely mechanical method, whereas meditation allows that energy to naturally arise from the fact that an empty mind no longer blocks its natural circulation.

This particular meditation of visualizing yourself as a set of bright white bones is called the white skeleton meditation, and more detailed instructions can be found in *Easy Meditation Lessons* (Bodri & Lee) and *The Little Book of Meditation* (Bodri).

One variant of this meditation method that is recommended for cancer patients, but which Meares did not study, is to visualize that your body flesh burns away by fire (rather than being stripped away), and then to visualize that your bones shine brightly as they are being burned and reduced to ashes. The next stage after becoming ashes is that the dust blows away and you just become dimensionless light. After awhile, you imagine that the light turns into vast empty space.

If you can do this, then at that time you are no longer holding onto any thoughts, just as Meares recommended. Thus you can achieve the recommended state of image-free mental freedom that is the same empty mind result that Meares called the "emptiness state."

There is yet another popular meditation method which you can practice that leads to the same result. You first imagine that your body becomes a giant silvery sun. After you have visualized being a bright silvery sun, you then imagine that you become boundless invisible light, and then let go of that imagination to let go of all thoughts and just remain in mental emptiness (quiet) without holding onto it. Once again you will then be cultivating an empty mental state free of most thoughts.

All these methods to assist the healing process have the one thing in common that Meares found effective. They help you quickly reach a state of cultivating mental emptiness, or the "absence of discriminative thought," which is the most powerful type of meditation practice possible for healing. It is more powerful than thought-filled meditation practices, such as guided imagery, which involve thinking throughout the entire meditation session and clinging to mental images all the way through. Instead, these practices only use visualization to first stabilize your mind of wandering thoughts. After your mind becomes stabilized, you then let go of those created images in order to simply abide in a quiet, peaceful mental zone. When your thoughts are quiet and mind is empty, your internal energy can then arise without mental obstructions and help open up your many acupuncture energy meridians. The resulting influx of healing energies throughout your body, because of meditation practice, can then help you feel better and assist you in beating cancer.

14
COFFEE ENEMAS FOR
LIVER DETOXIFICATION

If you have cancer, it is essential to eliminate as many toxic burdens from your life as possible because they all stand in the way of healing. Normally a "toxic burden" refers to various types of electromagnetic and chemical pollution, but as previously discussed this also includes burdens on your spirit and emotions.

Electromagnetic (EMF) pollution includes strong magnetic fields, dirty house electricity, microwave radiation and electromagnetic fields. All of these are known to produce illness, including certain types of cancers. Possible sources of strong EMF pollution inside the home or office include cell phones, wireless routers and poorly shielded electronic equipment such as laptops, computer screens, Wi-Fi stations, PCs, metering equipment etc. Because of the inverse square law, the power of these fields is reduced by the square of the distance from them. Therefore if you cannot do without them and cannot shield them or replace them with better alternatives, simply spend less time close to them.

Even more important than electromagnetic pollution is to eliminate as many toxic chemical burdens from your life as possible, many of which can cause cancer. The substances harmful to your body that you should avoid include fluoride and chlorine, chemical solvents and cleaners, lawn pesticides, insecticides, air fresheners, petrochemicals, tobacco, alcohol, and even unnecessary prescription drugs.

As a cancer patient, you should try to rid your house of all unnecessary chemical exposures from cosmetics to cleaning fluids to smelly chemicals, fabrics and carpets. Because of harmful paint fumes, do not undertake the repainting of your house at this time. Reduce toxic exposures to your body as much as possible. Throw everything away that you suspect is causing any allergies or sensitivities. Try to eat organic foods, too, to lower the burden of consuming pesticides and other chemical contaminants that your body cannot handle. The emphasis here is to reduce modern pollutants in your environment as much as possible.

The reason you should do this is that your liver and kidneys will already be taxed to the hilt from dealing with all the lysing debris produced by cancer therapies, so to prevent a detoxification overload, you want to be dealing with as few other chemical poisons to your body as possible. Just as you need to reduce the pathogenic load of microbes that threaten your immune system, you also need to reduce your toxic chemical load because remaining poisoned in any way will be a huge barrier to healing. As previously stated, Modifilan and other chelators can help detoxify your body of heavy metals and other poisons impacting your health. One of my favorite products along these lines is Nature's Pure Body Whole Body Program (NaturesPureBody.com).

Anyone who has gotten sick because of an accumulation of underlying toxicity needs to undergo various detoxification protocols to help remove that toxicity from the body. For some people, cancer quickly goes away after they remove the underlying cause of toxicity, such as any accumulation of carcinogenic poisons and heavy metals in the body, which then allows stronger cells to be built and more oxygen to enter the cells.

When you start to undergo most cancer therapies, the cancer cells within your body will start dying off and a massive amount of cellular debris will then be thrown into your bloodstream. All sorts of other toxins also get released during this process. Therefore, at the same time that you start getting better because your cancer starts breaking down, you will become internally toxic because your detoxification organs start becoming overloaded.

Your liver, kidney and other organs of detoxification will become strained as they try to keep up with this increasing load of poisons released into your system, and as they valiantly struggle to get rid of all the dead tumor toxins. Usually your liver and kidney filter out internal toxins without too many problems, but now these organs will get overloaded with all these burdens. They need some extra assistance to help to mobilize, neutralize and excrete all these toxins from your body.

This is why detoxification is a key cornerstone in many alternative medicine cancer protocols. It is also another reason why many people use fasting or juice fasting when they get cancer, and why they use nutritional or nutraceutical supplements to help with these issues.

One of the popular means to help your liver detoxify all these toxins is the at home practice of undertaking daily or weekly coffee enemas, first popularized by cancer treatment pioneer Dr. William Kelley and now used by many alternative, integrative physicians. A coffee enema stimulates your liver and is a great aid in elimination of the liver's toxic wastes. It is almost a certainty that a cancer patient can use extra help in stimulating their liver and there are few supplemental therapies better than a coffee enema for doing this.

Coffee enemas are not some new, weird detoxification therapy from left-field that was dreamed up by integrative physicians and alternative medicine doctors. They are very much mainstream, and have simply fallen out of favor over the years. They have actually been used in orthodox medicine by mainstream physicians *for over 50 years* to stimulate liver function and in turn, the processing and excretion of metabolic wastes from the body.

Coffee enemas are such a conventional medical treatment that the Merck Manual, which is the "Bible of the medical establishment," advocated coffee enemas as a liver stimulant in all editions from the first printing in 1898 on through to 1977! Coffee enemas were certainly in the conventional medical literature, and in fact were routinely recommended in nursing texts, too. Why? Because the liver is like a sponge that absorbs poisons and coffee enemas cause the liver to expel those toxins. They help drain the liver of poisons. Coffee enemas have been proven to help patients eliminate toxic waste material from the body and better deal with the burdens of detoxification.

The way it works is that the coffee's caffeine, taken rectally as an enema, basically sets up a reflex that stimulates nerves in the lower bowel and various detoxification pathways in the liver. Dr. Peter Lechner reports that the palmitic acid in the coffee promotes the activity of the glutathione S-transferase enzyme, which detoxifies the liver. It increases the activity of this enzyme by 600-700%, which is extremely useful to the body's detoxification needs since the blood circulates through the liver roughly five times during the time that the coffee enema is being held inside. Coffee enemas often result in great pain relief for cancer patients and many times a patient is able to reduce pain medication or get off of it completely through their usage.

If you have cancer, this is another supplemental therapy that you should consider doing at home and which does not interfere with any traditional mainstream cancer therapies.

A coffee enema is administered as follows.

- Add 3 tablespoonsful of fresh ground organic coffee to 1 quart of purified/distilled water. Do not use pre-ground coffee beans but grind the beans fresh. You should always use organic coffee that is caffeinated, never decaffeinated or the cheap instant coffee form the supermarket. Boil for 3-5 minutes to drive off the oils and then cover it with a lid and simmer for 15 minutes.
- Strain the coffee by passing it through gauze or an organic (non-bleached) coffee filter to remove large particles, and then allow it to cool to a comfortable body temperature. Never use it steaming hot. Put this in an enema bag that you hang elevated above you, whether you are standing, lying down and so on.
- Next lie down, lubricate the nozzle and insert it several inches into the rectum. Allow the coffee to drain very slowly into your intestines; use the clamp to adjust the speed of the flow. Relax and breath slowly while it goes into your intestine.
- Try to take in the whole bag and retain the coffee for around 15 minutes. If you feel spasms or unpleasant symptoms, close the clamp or lower the bag to the floor to stop the flow. Wait for half a minute and then try again. Sometimes gently massaging your belly will help you absorb more coffee.

- People who are ill may do this two or three times daily, or as needed. If you feel any immediate discomfort or experience a fever or headache, nausea, intestinal spasms and drowsiness, it generally indicates the successful flushing of toxins from your liver. You should increase the frequency of enemas if this happens because these symptoms indicate that you need more. You might try adding an extra enema at night before sleeping.
- After the last enema, you should inject about 50 ml of cold-pressed, organic sunflower seed oil, flaxseed oil or similar into your rectum to line your intestines and protect their mucus membranes.

A coffee enema sounds like a strange protocol only because you have to do it yourself and it is usually unfamiliar to most people. After you do it once, it is easy to do it again on a frequent basis. It just takes familiarity.

Countless integrative oncologists have found it so useful that it has been adopted as a standard practice by numerous cancer clinics all over the world. This is something you should consider doing at home to help yourself deal with conventional therapies and to help yourself get well.

There are also other therapies that can help you detoxify your liver, such as the equally famous liver-gall bladder flush. Many people offer commercial versions of this flush (ex. Herbdoc.com), and as with all these therapies, what you do or don't do to help detoxify your body is simply a sign of your commitment to beating cancer. The main liver cleansing therapy is the coffee enema, which is used by countless integrative physicians and global cancer clinics, and whose pedigree includes a prior history of common usage by mainstream medicine.

15
PROTOCOLS REQUIRING SUPERVISION

All the supplemental therapies covered can be easily done at home without any supervision. There are also many other very simple but extremely powerful integrative therapies available that can be done at home, but which require the ongoing supervision of a qualified health practitioner. The two major therapies along these lines, which you should know about, are cesium chloride and hydrazine sulfate therapies.

CESIUM CHLORIDE THERAPY

As you know, cancer cells are anaerobic and thrive in an acidic environment. One of the methods for attacking and beating cancer is to therefore increase the internal pH of cancer cells and change them to becoming more alkaline. The outer membranes of cancer cells are thick and hardened (which is why proteolytic enzymes are used in cancer therapies), often due to inflammation caused by toxins and carcinogens (which must be eliminated from the body through detoxification), which makes it difficult for oxygen to enter the cells while they take in glucose. Thus you can understand why Joanna Budwig formulated her FOCC mixture to help rebuild these cells. With these problems of getting oxygen into the cells, cancer cells then resort to fermenting glucose for energy instead of oxidizing it, and lactic acid is produced as a by-product. The acid reduces the pH within the cancer cell and overwhelms the normally controlled process of cellular replication with uncontrolled growth as a result. If you can break this acidity-based mechanism through some type of alkalization, you will then have yet another way of attacking cancer.

Many people know of this alkalizing pH theory for treating cancer because they have heard that there are baking soda cancer self-treatments, which you can readily find on Youtube. The idea is that you drink a "maple syrup and baking soda" mixture once a day right before you sleep as a cancer therapy. Because maple syrup is bonded with the baking soda, when the cancer cells take in the glucose of the maple syrup, the alkaline baking soda is also absorbed into the cells whereupon it weakens or destroys them. While this has been said to cure some people of cancer, this particular baking soda approach is not something you should rely upon because of various complexities. The principles of alkalizing cancer cells to kill them is a sound idea, but what is problematic is the particular approach you should take to put the principle into practice.

The idea of using sodium bicarbonate (baking soda) as a cancer treatment was greatly popularized by the Italian oncologist Dr. Tullio Simoncini. He developed his treatment plans after investigating whether alkalizing the body's pH to kill fungal infections would also treat cancer. If interested, you can find out more about Simoncini's controversial alkalizing protocols on his website or in his book, *Cancer is a Fungus*. This, too, is not a therapy to depend upon as a supplemental or primary cancer regimen; whether it is effective or not greatly depends on the type of cancer. However, there is a well-known alkalizing treatment for cancer, using cesium chloride, which has been proven to be quite effective for many types of cancers and has definitely saved thousands of people's lives.

It is simply a fact of science that tumor cells have a preference for absorbing alkaline minerals, such as cesium. All cells have an affinity for absorbing alkaline minerals because they resemble potassium. In particular, highly alkaline cesium has a special ability, which is that it can get into cancer cells when many other nutrients cannot. This is why radioactive cesium is used in cancer imaging systems to enter and thus identify cancerous cells.

Cesium targets cancer cells and does not enter healthy cells. When cesium gets into cancer cells, it increases the internal pH of the cells while the serum blood pH stays normal. This rise in alkalinity interrupts a cancer cell's metabolism so that it can no longer function, and then it simply dies off. Basically, the cesium limits the intake of glucose into the cell and without glucose, a cancer cell starves from lack of food, dies in a few days and is then eliminated by the body. The immune system can easily kill the starving, dysfunctional cancer cells once they have become damaged from responding to the cesium. Cesium also helps to neutralize the lactic acid produced by the cancer fermentation process.

When it enters cells, cesium not only kills cancer cells indirectly but it immediately halts cancer metastasis because it stops the cancer growth process. Thus it can start shrinking tumor masses within weeks.

If one subscribes to the microbial theory of cancer, it is also thought that the cesium entering cancerous cells might work to kill any cancer-causing microbes, reverting sick cells into normal cells. Whether or not you subscribe to this or any other explanation, it is unquestionably true that the cells that absorb enough cesium are "alkalized to the death" from the inside out. And even if you don't want to say that cancer can be cured through high pH alkalizing therapies, at the very minimum it is safe to say that cancer can *be controlled* using alkaline minerals. The truth, however, is that alkaline therapies *are an excellent systemic cancer treatment*, including for lymphomas or cancer metastasized to the bone.

Cesium chloride therapy can be used at any stage of cancer and can be used *with chemotherapy*. In fact, many people *need* to use high pH therapy together with chemotherapy, instead of alkalizing therapy alone, if they let their cancer progress too far without treatment or treatment success. Because cesium chloride therapy usually produces a speedy response it is perfect for fast growing cancers that are often highly fatal. Naturally, most patients make the mistake of waiting until their cancer progresses before using this therapy when they should get started on alkalizing therapies right away. In any case, even stage IV cancers, bone cancers and other cancers that have aggressively spread throughout the body usually respond to this treatment. Cesium chloride protocols are particularly favorable in cases of bone cancer and multiple myelomas because *the cesium can penetrate to the bone and bone marrow*. Being a mineral, cesium can even help protect the bones with these special cases of cancer.

Many people who have unsuccessfully used surgery, chemotherapy or radiation and who have been given only a short time to live, can often use cesium chloride therapy to immediately slow the spread of the cancer, shrink their tumors, reduce pain and buy time for other alternative protocols to work. Since it is a non-toxic approach that *targets cancer cells while leaving healthy cells alone*, the simplicity of the science makes you wonder why traditional oncologists don't use it more often. After all, it often eliminates cancer pain or reduces tumors faster than many other therapies. About the only major side effect is that patients taking cesium may experience some diarrhea or tingling of the lips and nose for about 20 minutes after using it.

A famous practitioner of cesium chloride cancer therapy was Dr. Hans A. Nieper, who practiced in Hannover, Germany, treating many American celebrities and executives, including Ronald Reagan. Because this treatment often causes swelling and inflammation due to the fact that the immune system starts attacking the dying cancer cells, it requires other supplemental protocols to be most effective, as well as a constant adjustment of dosages. For instance, your potassium levels should be monitored when you are on cesium therapy since it can also reduce your body's potassium levels. This is another reason why a physician should oversee its usage.

Cesium chloride therapy is a complex treatment with many restrictions and there is no single protocol that fits all cancer patients. Here's why. Since all cells have a potassium pump, they like to absorb potassium. Cesium, germanium, rubidium and lithium (alkaline minerals) all look like potassium to a cell, so if you take cesium and potassium at the same time it may lead to competition. On cesium therapy you therefore need to have frequent blood tests to see whether your potassium/sodium levels are getting out of balance because electrolyte imbalances often cause other health issues such as arrhythmia. This means that you need to work with an expert to use cesium chloride because a therapeutic protocol must be individually customized for each patient. It is difficult to find qualified experts for cesium therapy. Larry at Essense of Life (Essense-of-life.com) is one such expert who has been working with thousands of cancer patients, via telephone support, for many years and has extensive experience with cesium chloride.

When they subscribe to the idea of alkalizing cancer, patients often buy special water purifiers so that they can drink alkaline water, or start taking calcium supplements (such as coral calcium) to help neutralize the acidic pH within the body (which you should not combine with cesium chloride protocols since they are already an alkaline producer). Unfortunately, none of these approaches will break the thick protein shield around cancer cells that are usually attacked by proteolytic enzyme therapy. Cancer cells can only be killed when alkaline substances actually penetrate their membranes, and these therapies, while possibly helpful in various ways, certainly cannot produce cancer cures on their own.

HYDRAZINE SULFATE

As you know, cancer cells ferment glucose to get their energy, which in turn creates lactic acid as a waste product. This process makes cancer cells very acidic and the lactic acid produces pain in the body. The lactic acid travels through the bloodstream to the liver, which then uses an enormous amount of the body's energy to reconvert it back into glucose again. The recycled glucose is then, in turn, consumed once again as the food/fuel for increasing numbers of hungry cancer cells. As this cycle continues, a cancer patient starts to feel pain, becomes weaker and eventually wastes away, suffering from malnourishment because their glucose isn't reaching normal healthy cells.

Some patients also develop difficulties absorbing nutrients if their digestive system becomes damaged, which complicates this problem, or many cancer patients simply lose their appetite and stop eating because of their cancer. This is why many integrative cancer therapies try to feed non-cancerous cells (such as through highly absorbable supergreen powders) so that they stay healthy and an individual stays alive. Even then, cancer patients can still become malnourished because cancer cells, greedy for glucose, will absorb so much that regular cells will then starve. Cancer cells also need protein to make ATP for energy, and so people on low protein diets will often find their body raiding the protein stores of muscles and organs to get it. A cancer patient's body then wastes away to skin and bones from all these various reasons, which is a process called cachexia. This is why cancer patients often starve to death or experience organ failure before they can respond to their treatments.

While bodybuilders typically use D-Ribose, MSM and vitamin C to deal with lactic acid buildup in their muscles, hydrazine sulfate is one of the alternative treatments for cancer designed specifically to prevent cachexia. It interrupts the ability of the liver to convert lactic acid from tumors into glucose. By breaking the lactic acid cycle where it is converted back into glucose, this starves the tumors, inhibits their ability to metastasize and stops cachexia.

Dr. Joseph Gold, director of the Syracuse Cancer Research Institute, first proposed using hydrazine sulfate to combat cachexia in 1969. While doing research he came upon a reference to a chemical called hydrazine sulfate, which he realized could block a particular liver enzyme (the phosphoenol pyruvate carboxykinase enzyme, or PEP CK) necessary to convert lactic acid into glucose. He then reasoned that supplying hydrazine sulfate to the body could break the lactic acid cycle and thus inhibit the growth of cancer tumors while preserving normal healthy tissues. That's how it works: hydrazine sulfate blocks the cachexia cycle in the liver while cesium chloride blocks it within the cancer cells.

Dr. Gold's idea basically proposed *an entirely new means of non-toxic cancer chemotherapy* to break the pattern of starving healthy cells and vigorously growing cancer cells. In animal studies, he showed that hydrazine sulfate can stop glycogenesis in more than 50% of cancerous animals and because their sugar supply is cut off, their tumors begin to shrink.

In various independent clinical studies, including double-blind studies published in peer-reviewed medical journals, hydrazine sulfate's efficacy and safety has been *proven*. The only contrary results have come from the National Cancer Institute-sponsored trials of hydrazine sulfate which, for some unknown reason, purposefully used known incompatible agents with the test drug (medications that specifically neutralize the drug under study). Other than this one result, the great body of other research shows that hydrazine sulfate stabilizes tumors and significantly improves the nutritional status and survival of cancer patients. Patients who use it usually report a decrease in pain and better appetite, despite their cancer.

Whenever you have a case of patients who have lost their appetite due to their cancer or have become exceptionally weak, hydrazine sulfate should be considered. Because hydrazine sulfate does *not* kill cancer cells (and thus does not produce any cancer cell debris), it can be used with any other treatment, including chemotherapy (provided there is no conflict of allowed ingredients). Large scale trials suggest that it affects every type of tumor at every stage of cancer. Basically, if you want to stop cachexia then you can use hydrazine sulfate.

Hydrazine sulfate is inexpensive and has no severe side effects. However, there are many rules associated with using it safely and correctly (ex. you must avoid vitamin C, vitamin B-6, barbiturates, tranquilizers, sedatives, alcohol, morphine, antiemetics, etc.), so once again a patient should only use a hydrazine sulfate protocol by working with a knowledgeable expert. You should not use it as a self-treatment on your own, not because it doesn't work but rather because there is no standard safe dosage level and treatment regimen. Hydrazine sulfate is also difficult to use because there are many potential conflicts with other medications.

While the FDA and NIH have worked very hard to make hydrazine sulfate unavailable to the public, you can obtain hydrazine sulfate from Essense of Life (the cesium chloride vendor mentioned previously). To find the correct dosage for either your condition or a pet's condition, you should contact the Syracuse Cancer Research Institute for more information where you can also find out about potential conflicts with other medications.

As an interesting aside, the non-patentable chemical, dichloroacetate (DCA), has also been discussed as a possible cancer treatment option because it causes cancer cells to self-destruct by affecting the process of glycolysis. However, it uses a different mechanism than hydrazine sulfate. Because it is so inexpensive, I doubt that this substance will ever make it to mainstream usage but here are the particulars we know so far.

In our cells, there is an enzyme called pyruvate dehydrogenase kinase, or PDK, that regulates the flow of pyruvate into mitochondria. Pyruvate is necessary for glucose oxidation, which is the primary mechanism by which cells make energy. The energy requirements of cancer cells are very high since they grow so quickly. When the PDK enzyme is active, it forces cells to rely on glycolysis, which is the metabolic method that cancer cells use to supply their energy needs. If through some method you can suppress PDK, you can force a cancer cell to use glucose oxidation instead, which cancer cells do not prefer.

Dichloroacetate does exactly this – it suppresses PDK and forces a cancer cell to abandon its preferred metabolic process for producing energy. It also energizes mitochondria, which have sensors that react to biochemical abnormalities and which trigger a cell to self-destruct when they are found. Cancer cells grow so fast because the mitochondria are normally deactivated, but in this case DCA activates them again and thereby awakens their self-destruct capabilities. In essence, DCA flips a cancer cell's suicide switch back to "on" because it reactivates mitochondria that are the regulators of apoptosis (programmed cell death). Hence, DCA directly causes cancer cells to destruct and it works synergistically with other cancer therapies, such as radiation, gene therapy and viral therapy.

Are there other substances that induce cancer cell suicide? Ellagic acid, methylselenocysteine (selenium) and curcumin do. Curcumin, found in turmeric, can even inhibit thirty different inflammatory pathways to cancer by shutting off various cancer switches, so it is one of the strongest natural cancer preventatives (and curative aids) available. This is why it was recommended as an addition to your diet.

PAW PAW AND GRAVIOLA

There are many botanical substances that are effective when used as cancer treatments, but which are also difficult to use because they can interact with many other therapies. Graviola and Paw Paw (said to be stronger or more active than Graviola because of its more complex molecules) are two such botanicals.

These two botanicals are not listed as supplemental therapies because they should not be used with any other alternative cancer treatment due to potential conflicts. However, you might want to know something about them because they attack cancer in a different way than most other therapies. Rather than have two separate discussions, we will focus on Paw Paw, which is a cousin of the Graviola tree (also known as Guanabana and Soursop), since both have shown similar anti-cancer properties.

Paw Paw and Graviola are thought to work by slowing down or stopping the production of ATP inside cancer cells. This reduces the energy potential of a cancer cell to a low enough level that it can no longer process normal internal cellular processes, and then subsequently starves. For healthy non-cancerous cells the lower ATP production isn't much of a problem. However, because cancer cells must create energy from glucose by fermentation, ATP is much more critical for their survival because they require 10-17 times more energy than a normal cell. When the ATP energy level of a cell falls far enough, it basically starts to disintegrate, and this is how these botanicals attack cancer. Since the ATP production of all cells is reduced, however, one can start feeling tired when using these botanicals as a treatment.

Paw Paw works at ridding the body of cancer, but is slower than chemotherapy because its method of starving the cell of energy is a slower process than poisoning. In addition to this mechanism, Paw Paw also reduces the growth of blood vessels that nourish cancer cells, too, so it fights cancer via several different mechanisms.

Paw Paw has also been shown to kill multiple-drug resistant (MDR) cells, which are left behind after someone undergoes chemotherapy. When a person who was on traditional chemotherapy comes out of remission, a high percentage of their cancer cells are usually drug resistant cells. Most other mainstream or alternative cancer treatments don't show any effectiveness against multiple drug resistance, so the presence of MDR cancer cells would logically require the use of Paw Paw to treat these patients. This is something your doctor should investigate. Various agencies claim that it has no effectiveness against cancer at all and yet various studies show that it does. Paw Paw is one of the few therapies that can pass the blood-brain barrier, which is another reason to investigate its usage. Informal studies show that it is usually effective in about half of cancer cases.

The problem with both Paw Paw and Graviola is that they cannot be used with oxidative cancer treatments that raise cellular ATP and bolster cellular energy production. Therapies involving vitamin C, MSM/DMSO, hydrogen peroxide, colloidal silver, cesium chloride, glutamine, flax seed oil, Essiac tea and electro-medicine can nullify their effects. In other words, this would neutralize the potential of a lot of therapies, and to understand all the possible interactions would require the guidance of an expert!

Since they cannot be used with many integrative cancer treatments, even though they are synergistic with chemotherapy, they are not a highlighted protocol. They also carry the danger from lowering ATP and/or glutathione levels, so that normal healthy cells will lack the energy to protect themselves from internal microbial pathogens and opportunistic infections. In short, these botanicals may be hard to use and require the assistance of a skilled health practitioner to oversee the therapy. Nevertheless, they are easily researched on the internet.

LAETRILE (VITAMIN B17 OR AMYGDALIN)

Laetrile, which is found in apricot kernels and nearly 800 other plants, including in wheatgrass and raspberries (which also contain ellagic acid, as discussed), is another very famous anti-cancer compound. The story goes that after many years of research, the biochemist Dr. Ernst T. Krebs, Jr. isolated a new vitamin that he numbered B17 and named "laetrile."

Each molecule of laetrile contains the poison cyanide, which is tightly locked up with benzaldehyde and glucose. It was eventually discovered that the laetrile molecule reacts with an enzyme only found in cancer cells, beta-glucosidase, which cleaves off or "unlocks" the cyanide component of the molecule. When this happens, the cyanide is only released in the cancer cell, which then poisons the cell. This doesn't happen to normal healthy, non-cancerous cells because only cancer cells contain the unlocking enzyme beta-glucosidase.

When this cyanide unlocking occurs, the laetrile molecule also releases benzaldehyde at the same time. Benzaldehyde is another poison that acts synergistically with cyanide to help kill cancer cells. Therefore, laetrile uses two different methods for killing cancer cells. It also builds your immune system so that you can fend off future outbreaks of cancer. It reduces tumor pain in about half of cancer patients, and it is known for its ability to prevent metastasis for most types of cancer.

If an individual wanted to use laetrile as a primary cancer therapy, the amount required would require injections that are only available in non-U.S. cancer clinics, which typically administer it via an intravenous drip. This type of protocol is quite simple and said to be very effective if laetrile is used in high enough doses and combined with an effective diet and other supplemental therapies. However, this protocol requires expert technical support. In these clinics, the oncologists typically focus on a variety of factors such as rebuilding a patient's immune system and strengthening normal cells that have been weakened by other various cancer therapies.

Does laetrile work? You will find various researchers and agency organizations saying "no" and various non-U.S. doctors and clinics saying "yes." You can find studies attesting to its effectiveness in various books such *as Laetrile Case Histories: The Richardson Cancer Clinic (Dr. John Richardson), Alive and Well: One Doctor's Experience With Nutrition in the Treatment of Cancer Patients (Dr. Philip Binzel, Jr.)* and *World Without Cancer: The Story of Vitamin B17* (G. Edward Griffin) that can fill you in on the details of the molecule and its usage. You can watch the popular Youtube video of historian G. Edward Griffin's speech, "On the Science and Politics of Cancer," that also goes over the history of laetrile and how it has been suppressed by the pharmaceutical industry.

Like all the treatments we have discussed, you must understand that laetrile is not a magic cancer cure but just one type of natural therapy available in a naturopathic toolbox. You should never depend on it as the core of a cancer treatment or bet on this single therapy alone. It is just one possible component in what should be a total holistic regimen that requires serious diet, lifestyle changes and other cancer approaches addressing your whole body. In other words, it should certainly be combined with a number of other therapies in a total treatment protocol. Since it is not a therapy available in the U.S., only an oncologist outside the country could use it, so there is not much more to say other than to do your research if this particular adjunctive therapy interests you.

16
SOME SPECIAL THERAPIES
FOR PARTICULAR CANCERS

BREAST CANCER

If you have been diagnosed with breast cancer, an essential part of a permanent cure lies in removing any root canals in your mouth.

No matter how hard a dentist tries to disinfect the inside of the tooth after the root canal has been cleaned out, there is no way to eliminate it entirely. Root canals always harbor hidden infections and these have been directly linked to cancer or other degenerative diseases. The evidence is overwhelming that dead teeth left in the mouth become toxin factories that produce illness at locations other than at the tooth. You can read *Root Canal Cover-Up* (George Meinig), *The Roots of Disease: Connecting Dentistry and Medicine* (Kulacz and Levy) and *Uniformed Consent: The Hidden Dangers in Dental Care* (Huggins and Levy) for more information on this.

A variety of researchers in biological dentistry have found a clear connection between breast cancer and root canals on the very teeth that share the same acupuncture meridians as the breast tumor, which are usually molars. In other words, when you have breast cancer there is a high likelihood that you have had a root canal on one of your molars, specifically the one which is smack on the acupuncture meridian that leads to the cancerous tumor.

If you have root canals and breast cancer, many integrative oncologists will therefore tell you to "remove the dead teeth" or warn that you will not get rid of a possible source of the problem. Dr. Josef Issels of Germany, who had one of the highest cancer cure rates in history after 40 years of treating over 16,000 cancer patients, insisted that *all his patients* have their root canals removed. He had found that over 97% of his cancer patients had received root canals (while Dr. Rau at the Paracelsus clinic in Switzerland had found over 90%) and so he made their removal *mandatory* before he would begin his cancer treatments. Other researchers have confirmed his findings that a large majority of breast cancer patients have had root canals (or some other dental involvement) in the very teeth that lie on acupuncture meridians to the affected breast. Some health practitioners even say that at least 50% of cancer's reversal lies in the mouth!

Here's what many researchers report that they often find. If you have a root canal on a tooth connected with the gall bladder meridian, you might end up feeling gall bladder pain. In other words, the root of the problem is in your tooth rather than gall bladder, which is why gall bladder surgery often does not remove pain in that organ. If you have a root canal on a tooth connected with another organ, you might develop illness or pain in that organ system, too. Researchers are finding this connection, which is a basic tenet of traditional Chinese medical theory, over and over in their investigations.

Many explanations have been offered as to why chronic infections in root canals contribute to cancer (see also *The Roots of Disease: Connecting Dentistry and Medicine* by Kulacz and Levy, and *Uniformed Consent* by Huggins and Levy). The most popular idea is that various pathogenic microbes gain a foothold in a devitalized tooth and its three miles of micro-canals. There they reproduce with succeeding anaerobic generations becoming more and more toxic due to the lack of oxygen conditions. Eventually as their numbers grow, the toxic effects of these microbes start appearing along the acupuncture meridian routes that touch their point of origin in the mouth. This somehow sets the stage for cancer.

The evidence from so many studies and integrative oncologist findings is clear: to get over breast cancer *you should get rid of your root canals* in order to clear up the infections. If you are diagnosed with breast cancer, you must always look to remove the root contributing causes of the condition. While some of the other possible causes behind breast cancer include the use of aluminum antiperspirants, xenoestrogens, living too close to a nuclear power plant facility, wearing a bra, or undergoing too many breast x-rays, having root canals is near the top of this list of possible causes.

Some experts say that the medical radiation exposure from breast exams is probably the single most important cause behind the breast cancer epidemic because one mammogram is equivalent to the ionizing radiation from one thousand chest x-rays. The "low energy" X-rays used in mammograms were also found to cause approximately four times, and as much as six times more mutation damage than higher energy X-rays. If you think there are early screening benefits to X-ray breast exams, which the mainstream claims, you should rethink this conclusion because study after study show that these benefits are simply not there at all. On the other hand, there is the cumulative cancer risk from yet another event of intense radiation exposure. In short, mammograms are not recommended for women under fifty years of age unless they have unusual risk factors for cancer.

Some types of breast cancer are also just "benign lesions" that end up being over-diagnosed and over-treated, so you must be aware of this if breast cancer is your diagnosis. Furthermore, the likelihood of being diagnosed with a false positive over ten years is over 50% for women who undergo annual breast screening. On top of this, according to Dr. Susan Love of UCLA, at least 30% of tumors found by mammograms go away all on their own when you do nothing at all, meaning an aggressive response is often an over-reaction. You should consult Breastcancerchoices.org for more details on these various issues before you pursue overly aggressive therapy.

What else should you know?

A pioneering study in Israel even found that breast cancer rates dramatically declined after pesticides were banned from dairy production. Israeli breast cancer rates used to be among the highest in the world until Israeli women demanded that the country ban carcinogenic pesticides that were contaminating milk and dairy products. In the decade afterwards, breast cancer incidents for women aged 24-34 declined by 34%, while rates in other countries increased, once again proving the role that pesticides play in cancer. This study, and others, re-iterates the need for clean food in your diet and the need to use various detoxification routines for health.

Vitamin D is another substance extremely important for helping to prevent and fight breast cancer. Iodine is also helpful as well (see *Breast Cancer and Iodine: How to Prevent and How to Survive Breast Cancer* by Dr. David Derry). Many people have beaten cancer with iodine supplementation alone, and it is often used to massage the breast to eliminate breast cysts. CoQ10 (Jarrow brand Q-Absorb), at doses of 100-400 mg/day, have also been used with metastatic breast cancer. CoQ10, D-ribose and ATP are common parts of other cancer treatment protocols simply to help patients have more energy and help prevent cachexia.

Several studies have also found a linkage between wearing bras and breast cancer. The standard advice is that if you want to wear a bra, you should purchase a bra without a metal support wire to help prevent breast cancer. In a world of increasing EMF pollution bombarding us all day long from every possible angle, the metal support wire is thought to act like a receiving antenna for harmful electromagnetic radiation and it is placed right on top of the breast.

Whatever therapies you choose to undergo for breast cancer, it is imperative that you use detoxification routines and nutritional therapy as part of your overall protocol for getting well. With enough integrative cancer therapies it is sometimes possible to avoid a mastectomy entirely. It may therefore be prudent to do some careful research of your various options upon hearing you have breast cancer rather than immediately rush into a mastectomy.

Alternative or integrative treatments for breast cancer are often more effective than conventional therapies, less expensive and offer alternatives to surgery and chemotherapy, without the long-term recovery time needed after conventional treatments are used. There is even compelling evidence which suggests that a nutritional approach to post-operative breast cancer treatment far exceeds in safety and effectiveness any regimen of chemotherapy and radiation that is traditionally used in hospitals. Part of the nutritional therapy principles includes avoiding soy foods, since they can make breast cancer grow faster.

Now as to mastectomies (or even hysterectomies in cases of cervical cancer), before you immediately rush into surgery to lose a breast, you have to consider that a change in the size of a tumor has very little to do with either a cancer patient's survival or their quality of life. You will have to change something internally to get rid of the conditions that caused cancer, rather than just cut out a tumor or try to radiate it away. Many integrative physicians strive to do just that while leaving the tumor alone and simply watch it shrink through their efforts. They can often help breast cancer (or cervical cancer) go into remission without a woman needing to lose her breasts, lymph nodes, uterus and so on. There is a saying that "If the cancer doesn't get you, then the radiation and chemo will," and they try to help women avoid this becoming an actuality.

Cutting a breast off through a mastectomy (or cutting out the uterus or any other organ) therefore does not solve the problem of cancer. As the very least, a woman *should consider a less invasive lumpectomy rather than mastectomy*, and she will have to look for an expert surgeon who has done this as a matter of course. If she undergoes surgery, she will also still have to change her diet and lifestyle and adopt all sorts of supplemental treatments that can help change her inner terrain and remove the conditions that caused cancer in the first place. I agree with Burton Goldberg that if you get breast cancer you should consider an integrative oncologist if you want to save your breasts. You should understand what your options are, visit a biological dentist, avoid sugar and change your diet and pay attention to your immune system.

A last point is that if you are to undergo breast surgery, you should consider scheduling your surgery after ovulation (in the second half of the menstrual cycle), since some studies show that this tends to produce better outcomes. Many researchers believe that operations during the luteal phase produced "significantly better prospects," perhaps because the protective benefit of progesterone during that phase helps to balance what had been estrogen dominance. Either this special timing matters or it doesn't matter at all, in which case it certainly doesn't hurt to err on the side of caution, since it may even extend your life. You can reference Dslrf.org for details about the 32 studies that have evaluated this factor.

BRAIN CANCER

If the issue is a brain tumor, you should look into the antineoplaston approach of Dr. Stanislaw Burzynski, which has been successful with some of the most difficult forms of cancer, including childhood brain melanomas. It is available at the Burzynski Clinic in Houston, Texas. A movie about his innovative cancer approach is available on the internet entitled "Burzynski, the Movie; Burzynski: Cancer is Serious Business." It is also available at BurzynkiMovie.com and the Whitakerhealthfreedom.com website.

For an oncologist who has cured countless cancer cases, which is a proven fact, Dr. Burzynski has certainly felt the pressure of incredible legal harassment from the FDA, which illustrates why most oncologists will rarely use anything other than mainstream approved cancer treatments. The story of the Hoxsey formula (which can be seen in the videos "Cancer: The Forbidden Cures" and "Hoxsey: How Healing Becomes a Crime") and the story of Dr. Andrew Ivy's persecution by the FDA for promoting an unorthodox cancer therapy, both illustrate similar lessons about the risks of federal persecution for those who offer effective non-mainstream approaches against cancer. Burzynski is fighting this same battle despite his track record of curing the incurable.

If you have any type of brain tumor or brain cancer, you should also immediately stop using a cell phone until you can rule out that the powerful EMFs (electromagnetic fields) entering your brain from your cell phone have not contributed to your condition. Without a doubt, extensive exposure of cell phone radiation to the head definitely causes brain tumors, and you don't want to be using cell phones when fighting brain cancer if you are one of the individuals most sensitive to this type of radiation. Either switch to a different low-EMF cell phone model, use some EMF radiation reduction methods, or eliminate cell phone usage entirely. Industry officials will sometimes say that there is no linkage between brain cancer and cell phone usage, but you always have to exercise your thinking muscles to penetrate through the claims of public relations.

In industries where huge amounts of money are at stake (and litigation lawsuits), many scientific studies indicating a link between the industry's products and health conditions are usually debunked by the industry or by the scientists who are funded by the industry. This is a common enough story seen time and again on investigative television programs like *60*

Minutes, so you have to do your own research to confirm whether there is a linkage between cell phone usage and brain tumors, and then draw your own conclusions.

A naturopathic-nutritionist colleague of mine told me a story, which happened several years ago, of a brain surgeon who was wondering why he was now seeing so many patients with tumors in the exact same region of the brain. One day, he saw one of his physician colleagues running down the hospital hallway switching his cell phone from ear to ear as he was talking, and then the answer immediately dawned upon him. The location of the tumors he was seeing were even matched with whether the patients were left or right-handed when holding their cell phones against their heads.

The short of it is this: if you are a heavy cell phone user and get brain cancer, it is probably contributing to your condition. If that is the case, if you don't stop using your cell phone then you are likely to lose your life. If you are placing a strong radiation source right next to your head, you are certainly risking the development of brain tumors. So it is your choice whether or not you should continue using a piece of technology that is known to produce tumors in the brain.

It is a fact that prolonged exposure to EMFs can definitely cause cancer. According to one recent research finding from Brazil that adds to the list of growing evidence, even the weaker exposure to radiation from cell phone towers could be attributed to over 7,000 cancer deaths. For example, in Belo Horizonte, Brazil's third largest city, it was found that over 80% of those who succumbed to certain types of cancer resided within approximately a third of a mile from one of the many cell phone antenna in the city. This study does not stand alone by itself; the closer you live to a broadcasting antennae, the greater your contact with strong electromagnetic fields and the greater your dangers from prostate, breast, lung, kidney and liver cancer, which are the cancers most associated with exposure to electromagnetic fields (EMFs).

Day by day, all of us are becoming exposed to stronger doses of microwave radiation, magnetic fields, "dirty house electricity" and EMF pollution, which can cause health problems such as cancer in many individuals who are particularly sensitive. To reduce this growing daily exposure and lower your cancer risks from all types of radiation, you might choose to use some of the devices at TooMuchEMF.com, which summarizes the most popular and effective products for reducing harmful EMF exposure.

Brain cancer is one of the trickiest types of cancer to treat, particularly because of the dangers of swelling in the brain. Because swelling is a concern, a patient should ask their physician to consider sulfur DMSO/MSM therapies, which will penetrate the blood-brain barrier and help keep down any swelling inside the brain. You might also consider adding turmeric/curcumin to the diet (in doses taken throughout the day) since it is a potent anti-inflammatory and anti-cancer agent. A person with brain cancer should use as many immune system building therapies as possible because the white blood cells and other immune components created by these treatments are guaranteed to get past the blood-brain barrier.

SKIN CANCER

Your skin is one of the main organs of elimination for your body. If you have skin cancer, you must ask yourself, "What is happening *internally* that I have developed skin cancer?" Skin cancer is often signaling that there is a need for a full body detoxification and tremendous dietary changes to get well.

Three alternative medicine salves or ointments are commonly used to treat skin cancer. These are "Cansema Black Topical Salve" (also known as black salve), "PDQ! Herbal Skin Cream," and "BEC-5 Curaderm Cream."

The BEC-5 cream is an amazing product, invented by a physician. You might know it by its other popular name, "Curaderm." BEC-5 is an extract of solasodine glycoside (found in eggplant and Devils' Apple weed), which binds to cancer cells and causes them to rupture, while leaving healthy cells alone. In other words, it penetrates and kills cancer cells, but not healthy normal skin cells. It was discovered by Dr. Bill Cham on the island of Vanuatu, when he found that local farmers were rubbing the "Devil's Apple" plant onto the backs of animals that were experiencing skin cancers. These farmers were having considerable success in its removal.

Since its commercial introduction, it has cured over 70,000 skin cancer cases in Australia. Even the Royal London Hospital found that it cured nearly 80% of skin cancer cases in a placebo-controlled trial. One study of 72 patients showed a 100% cure rate within 13-weeks of applying BEC-5, although it usually works quicker than that. You can readily purchase it via the internet and apply it on your own, which is great since most doctors won't even know about it. It is simple to use, has no adverse side effects, incredibly inexpensive and works nearly every time (on squamous and basal cell cancers even as large as two to three inches).

While some people have reportedly resolved cases of melanoma and squamous cell skin cancer in a few weeks just by spraying the lesions twice a day with colloidal platinum, gold and silver, the BEC-5 is a more tested and proven treatment option. You can read more about its main ingredient in Dr. Bill Cham's *The Eggplant Cancer Cure* and *Inspired by Nature, Proven by Science.*

BONE CANCER

For bone cancer patients, many of the best alternative cancer therapies involve mineral-based treatments because bone is basically composed of minerals. Cesium chloride, being a mineral-based treatment, is a possibility that can help protect the bones, so it is a supplemental treatment you should strongly consider. Another product to look into is clodronate, which stops breast cancer from spreading to the bones. Unfortunately, it is not available in the United States.

Limu juice should also be considered as a supplemental therapy for bone cancer patients, and if the bone cancer is related to radiation exposure, a MSM/DMSO protocol should be considered because sulfur is implicated as a healing agent in many radiation caused illnesses.

17
SUMMARY AND CONCLUSIONS

Cancer feeds on glucose, which comes from sugar. It thrives in an acidic environment rather than an alkaline environment. It thrives in anaerobic conditions, meaning without oxygen. Cancer cells have unusually thick cellular membranes. It also proliferates when your immune system is weak and when your DNA replication process has gone haywire for some reason.

All these facts provide hints as to how you can help beat cancer and heal yourself so it permanently stays away, using therapies other than chemo, radiation and surgery that do not address its causes. A tumor is just a symptom of the disease, so cancer is telling you that you are biochemically imbalanced and need to systemically readjust your body's internal biochemistry to eliminate all the possible systemic causes of the condition. If you do not do this, then even if you get well it is likely to come back.

You can think of cancer as like the unwanted algae which starts to grow in a swimming pool. When the pH of a swimming pool drops (so that it becomes acidic) and the pool chemicals become out of balance, the favorable environment will cause the algae to start growing out of control. If you want to get rid of the algae, you need to raise the pH of the water, rebalance the chemicals and then the algae will die off naturally. Once the algae starts dying, you can then vacuum the debris out of the pool. In a similar way, you can use all sorts of therapies to change your internal biochemical terrain, kill cancer and help detoxify your body of all the cellular lysing debris that is produced when cancerous cells start dying.

All chronic degenerative health conditions require that you rebalance your inner terrain to create an environment that supports health and healing. Therefore with cancer, you cannot just undergo surgery, radiation and chemo and expect that you have created the conditions whereby you will get well. With cancer remission and survival rates so low, this idea stretches the bounds of common sense, which is why I wrote this book to help you with supplemental therapies to attack this issue of imbalanced biochemistry.

Beating cancer is not solely about killing cancer cells, although that is the most popular mainstream approach to the problem. It's not just about fixing DNA replication problems, killing pathogenic microbes to lower your immune burdens or detoxifying your body of poisons. It is about correcting *all these conditions* and other unbalanced aspects of your internal biochemistry, because if you don't address the underlying systemic problems that have contributed to causing cancer in the first place, then the chances are that cancer won't truly go away, or will just keep returning.

To treat cancer you should be working at systemically correcting your body's biochemistry. You must go after this problem from different angles to maximize your chances of a permanent cure, which is why we have included many different supplemental therapies. The field of electro-medicine and bio-oxidative therapies were left out because they are complicated subjects that deserve entire books on their own to weave through the products that lack credibility. Basically, if you work with nutrition, supplements and other complementary therapies to create an environment where cancer cannot survive, then you have a good chance of eliminating it entirely. All these supplemental strategies help to create that environment. Don't just depend on chemo, surgery and radiation to get well but work to change your internal terrain.

This idea of rebalancing your body is an ages old medical principle but today's current medical system often ignores this timeless wisdom. It goes after the symptoms of cancer with a vengeance but doesn't bother to work at correcting the accumulation of numerous damaging factors and underlying systemic conditions that brought it about. This is why many people never get well, or their cancer returns. It is also why many people who bother to think about these matters start using extra integrative therapies and supplemental protocols to help adjust their bodies so that they can rid themselves of cancer for good.

As to your diet, what you should and should not eat if you get cancer is a very big question because this is very important, too. Your diet may be the single most important issue to your getting well and beating cancer or not.

There are many special diets that fight cancer, but you must pick the right one for yourself otherwise you simply won't follow it. Along these lines, what you *don't eat* is often more important than what you do eat because you must switch from eating unhealthy junk foods to eating "clean foods" packed with healthy nutrition.

To recap on the basic anti-cancer diet, here's what you should avoid. You must get off all forms of sugar. You must also reduce your intake of simple carbohydrates including white bread, pasta, rice, refined grains and other foods that transform into glucose quickly through the process of digestion. Honey and molasses should also be avoided except when they are employed in specific protocols that use them in a controlled fashion. Don't use artificial sweeteners either, and stop drinking soda and alcohol. Stay away from highly processed foods with a lot of chemicals and artificial preservatives (so avoid MSM and food additives). Avoid milk and dairy unless they are specifically used in a cancer therapy. Avoid bad oils and trans fats, such as margarine and fried foods. Avoid foods that might contain fungus, such as peanuts and cashews.

To clean up your diet you should eat organic foods as much as possible. You may or may not consume meat depending on the specific diet you are using, but if you are a meat-eater you should eat free range, grass fed meat along with digestive supplements, but you should avoid pork. Eliminate all GMO foods, since they can cause tumors and organ damage, and all foods to which you are allergic or have a sensitivity. You should also avoid chlorine and fluoride in your drinking and bathing water.

You should also add to your diet beneficial foods known to have cancer-killing ingredients, such as asparagus and broccoli (and the cruciferous vegetables). Try to add fresh wheatgrass juice, barley grass juice and carrot juice to your diet (any daily anti-cancer vegetable/fruit juicing routine) to which you can add some sort of extra supergreens powder that contains many cancer-fighting ingredients. You should be drinking fresh vegetable juices two to three times per day. Since the body needs protein to build healthy new cells, when vegetarian look for supergreen products containing spirulina since it contains plant-based protein, or hemp protein that contains all the essential amino acids. To this powder I would add a scoop of any raspberry/berry powder containing ellagic acid because of its anti-cancer benefits. One additional nutritional powder to consider is Cellect, which is a key ingredient in many cancer fighting nutritional protocols. You can easily mix it with fresh fruit and vegetable juices.

The Budwig cottage chess-flaxseed oil combination should also be added to your diet because it will help you build healthy new cells, but don't take it within 1.5 hours of Cellect or any supergreens formula. You can combine the use of the Budwig protocol and Cellect by following the instructions at CellectBudwig.com. This combination will start working very quickly in protecting your body's healthy cells while attacking cancer cells, but it won't create any kind of inflammation or swelling. It works to create an inner terrain that will stop the spread of the cancer, and can even be used with chemotherapy. The raw vegetable juices, supplemented by supergreen powders, will especially help along these lines.

Is it reasonable that a doctor might say to you, "No, starting now you cannot eat healthy. You cannot eat cottage cheese and flaxseed oil, or nutritional powders known to cure cancer that will make you stronger."? If you hear that eating healthy clean foods, which you probably have not been doing your entire life, will now interfere with your cancer treatments, you better reevaluate the doctor who is treating you. If you hear that nutritional supplements are now a no-no, you better seek a cancer physician who is more up-to-date with the research. This will quite often be a physician familiar with holistic/naturopathic healing methods and their proven track record in cancer treatments.

With cancer, you need help with your immune system, too. Whether pathogenic microbes can really cause cancer or not, you will still want to reduce your internal pathogenic burden when you get cancer so that your immune system is freed up to be able to fight it. Doing so will also reduce/prevent opportunistic infections that commonly occur to cancer patients, so the simplest way to accomplish these goals is to use colloidal silver and various immune boosting supplements, like transfer factor, to help.

What are you going to drink? No longer should it be soda, milk or other sweet drinks. You should consider drinking tea, namely green tea, Pau d'arco tea and Essiac tea. There is also the anti-cancer drink, Limu juice, and of course various nutrient rich juices such as wheatgrass, barley grass and carrot juice, which can be supplemented with supergreen powders. Remember that carrot juice is a cancer cure in itself and you should never fear its sugar content. Barley grass and wheatgrass powder/juice are also of notice because they contain many anti-cancer nutrients. Because of their enzyme content they are considered a type of full-spectrum enzyme support for healing. They will help your body with its task of detoxification while you are trying to heal.

There are even juicing diets, such as the Gerson diet, which depend on drinking vegetable/fruit juices that are very high in anti-cancer nutrients. You shouldn't worry that these juices contain too much sugar when they are used as part of a well-planned healing protocol. As stated, to these juices you can add specific nutritional powders that contain ingredients known to help you heal.

Whether or not you use juices, you should supplement your diet with various powders that may be helpful in various ways, such as supergreen foods, ellagic acid, glutamine powder, Cellect and so on. You should also add the Budwig flaxseed oil and cottage cheese combination to your diet (for solid mass tumors or less advanced cancers) since it will bring new life to your body and its cellular processes, attacking cancer tumors and building stronger new cells in response. If you are helping yourself at home, start with a better diet, add the Budwig FOCC mixture to your daily routine and a special shake/smoothie of fresh vegetable juices and green food nutritional powders according to your considerations. You should be consuming a fresh vegetable juice/supergreen powder combination several times per day.

There are several reasons to also start using enzymes to help digest your meals, or proteolytic pancreatic enzymes on an empty stomach to help digest cancer cells. Almost every integrative cancer physician recommends enzymes because they strip away the thick protein coatings around cancer cells, which then allows your immune system to finally recognize them as dysfunctional so that it can destroy them.

Your doctors, whether they are mainstream or integrative physicians, can guide you through the various therapies they use to treat cancer. However, only a doctor who is holistically or naturopathically oriented, which we commonly call an integrative, alternative or complementary physician, is likely to teach you about these extra supplemental therapies you can use at home that easily and safely complement most mainstream orthodox treatments.

It's not that a mainstream oncologist will deliberately withhold information on these therapies. Most of them don't know anything at all about these methods because they lack sufficient education (they often are only taught the trio of chemotherapy, surgery and radiation by medical school), and so they think they are doing you a favor telling you to run away from these proven helpmates, often calling it "quackery." Often they do know something about these proven approaches and their effectiveness, but they may want to remain silent to keep their licenses and stay away from federal legal problems, which they assume will be used to harass them if they use these. You, as a free human being, who is potentially dying, have the legal opportunity to use many various supplemental therapies that might help your condition. You simply must do some careful research, decide whether you want to do so and then find skilled health experts who can help guide you.

What can you use? We only went over just a very few therapies, but they are the *most powerful simple ones* that can be safely used alongside most mainstream therapies while attacking cancer from different perspectives. For supplemental help that targets cancer from the angle of DNA replication there are the Beljanksi formulas and colloidal platinum (in Meso-SGPS). From the angle of immune assistance there is colloidal silver (in Meso-SGPS), naltrexone, Carnivora, *Nerium oleander* extract, and many other nutraceutical products. Various botanical preparations that in some way attack cancer directly include Carnivore, *Aloe arborescens*, *Nerium oleander*, Limu juice and Essiac tea. We also have green tea and Pau d'arco tea that have strong cancer fighting abilities and which are extremely easy to add to a daily diet. We did not cover products like Oncolyn or Tian Xian due to potential complications, but these are also possible cocktails of beneficial plant extracts that fight cancer. To help prevent metastasis and/or angiogenesis there are ellagic acid, colloidal gold (in Meso-SGPS) and Dr. Rath's easy amino acid protocol. There are also supplements or therapies that help detoxify your body. It is extremely easy to add any of these supplements to a daily routine since they usually involve swallowing a few capsules or drinking a few cups of liquid per day. That's how simple it is to use them.

As stated, taking pancreatic proteolytic enzymes will also help dissolve away the thick protein coating of cancer cells, so that the immune system will find it easier to recognize these cells and chemotoxic agents can more easily enter them. Cesium chloride will alkalize cancer cells from the inside out so that cancer cell metabolism becomes dysfunctional, while hydrazine sulfate will cut down on cancer pain. These are just a few chosen supplemental therapies, but they are core treatments used by many highly successful integrative cancer oncologists and clinics. The beauty is that you can use them at home alongside of most conventional cancer therapies, or just use them alone, as long as you receive expert advice and guidance.

As you can see, there are all sorts of supplemental therapies available to help you. Some therapies will help your normal cells stay strong and thus keep you alive while other therapies start to work. Some therapies will slow down the spread of cancer or halt it. Some therapies will directly attack cancer and try to destroy it. Some therapies will try to repair cancerous cells and revert them back to normal. Some therapies will deal with nutritional deficiencies that might be related to cancer. Some will try to correct problems with DNA replication. Some will work on angiogenesis. Some will help reduce the acidity of cancer cells or lower their ATP energy so they are weakened. Some will build stronger cell membranes and help increase the oxygen uptake by cancer cells. Some will work on activating apoptosis (programmed cell death) or phagocytosis. Some therapies will help rebuild your immune system and deal with opportunistic infections.

Many therapies other than our basic "super cancer fighters" are available (such as laetrile, Paw Paw, etc.) but we have only emphasized those that don't normally require a doctor's supervision or conflict with other supplemental therapies. To use those treatments it is always best to work with a physician or expert cancer coach who has years of cancer experience and knows about the stages of progress and possible interactions. A physician can also administer the extremely valuable bio-oxidative therapies or intravenous therapies, and you should look into electro-medicine therapies as well. Modern electrodermal screening equipment, such as used by an **Asyra Pro** practitioner, can use electronic resonance to help differentiate between which supplements or therapies you should avoid and which ones will probably help you. With hundreds of options out there, having any means to select the most beneficial supplements or therapies for your personal condition, and weed out what is useless, is priceless. Since the Asyra device can detect heavy metals, chemicals, bacteria, viruses, herbicides, hormonal problems or nutrient deficiencies that are affecting the body and which might play a role in cancer, this type of screening to help you decide on a course of action is well worth your time.

If you are doing any of this on your own, you should always ask experts about any potential conflicts between these and traditional therapies, and any side effects for your own special situation. Research everything, ask questions of experts (keeping potential conflicts of interest in the back of your mind, such as whether they make money from something they recommend), and then decide accordingly. Read books, research articles on the internet, and talk to experts and other cancer survivors. Try to find someone, such as an integrative physician or experienced cancer coach, to help you navigate through all the options that mainstream medicine won't talk about.

It is *your life at stake* and with the risks so high, wisdom would suggest that you do everything possible to get healthy and you should start right away. This requires you to recognize the laws and various conflicts of interest that would prompt doctors and hospitals to recommend only their "approved" approaches over others. You have read the research findings and clinical results from many rock solid doctors who might offer very successful alternatives to the mainstream therapies.

If you are reading this, you already recognize that you must assume some responsibility for helping to heal your condition. When anyone looks at the cancer cure rates, they will quickly realize that cancer patients can spend hundreds of thousands of dollars on orthodox treatments that may do nothing except weaken their body and allow their condition to spread, while emptying their wallet. Many of those same patients, lacking wisdom, will complain that they must spend a few hundred dollars a month on alternative therapies *that can be thirty times more effective than orthodox treatments!* These might save their life where the mainstream therapies might fail them.

The medical establishment is quite content to use treatment regimens that have a 5-year cure rate of just 2-3%, and it is a common story that uninformed patients will easily spend so much money on these mainstream therapies that afterwards they cannot afford the most effective natural treatments available. They usually turn to them only AFTER their body has been severely damaged by the mainstream protocols, which lowers their chances of success. This is why you should get started on supplemental therapies *right away* for at the very minimum they might help you protect yourself from such devastation.

Integrative treatment plans designed and overseen by a health expert often have a 90% chance of eliminating cancer if a patient gets started on the alternative medicine pathway immediately, but the media does not seem to care about cure rates enough to popularize these results so that everyone knows this. Like most profit seeking organizations, it really cares about who has the most money to pay for advertisements and what is most profitable for the media organization, rather than what is righteous.

There is no therapy within this book that you should consider a "cancer cure." While some of these therapies have beaten cancer on their own, they are all *adjunctive therapies* and you must do a lot of such simultaneous things to get well. Nevertheless, you must also understand that there is a loud chorus of legitimate patients who have cured themselves through alternative avenues to the mainstream cancer treatments, and it is totally up to you to determine how much to rely on any particular therapy or cancer treatment. If the treatment itself is killing you or destroying your quality of life, you really must rethink it.

One last bit of advice: cancer is a complicated subject, so don't try to cure yourself at home without the supervision and guidance of a physician. These are just introductions to adjunctive therapies meant to *supplement* a skilled doctor's care and treatment. Therefore, use all the information you learn from all the sources available *together with an appropriate health professional* to get started at combining several highly effective cancer treatments together. Your life is at stake, so your job is to find the clinics, physicians, and other health professionals who will be most helpful to helping you get well. You know with 100% certainty what your outcome will be if you do nothing at all, so it is only by taking a proactive approach that you can change that outcome for the better.

The final approach you use does not have to exclude mainstream therapies, which are often the most effective available, but it also should allow leeway for some of the helpful supplemental therapies discussed that you might use at home. With just the handful of supplemental therapies mentioned in this book, skillfully applied with the help of a knowledgeable health practitioner, you should be able to supercharge your other cancer treatments and improve your condition tremendously. While mainstream thinking is usually centered around the idea of treating tumors rather than the body's overall health condition, most of these supplemental therapies take a different approach because they assume that a systemic condition develops first *and then* the cancer. By addressing the body as a whole, while mainstream treatments typically focus on tumors, they easily supplement most mainstream cancer treatments quite nicely.

Nothing works 100% of the time, so combining several proven synergistic therapies together, which have individually cured cancer in some cases and simultaneously attack it from different angles, is a reasonable way to achieve a better quality of life, longer life, and outsmart your cancer that might be impossible to attain using just mainstream therapies alone. You should choose your supplemental therapies with care, just as you should choose your oncologist with care, and I hope that these proven natural therapies can help you get started in that direction.